DAVID CARRADINE'S
TAI CHI
WORKOUT

David Carradine's career began in acting. Having appeared
in Broadway plays, he then migrated to Hollywood, where
he pursued a career in film and television leading to his role
in the highly successful series *Kung Fu*. He lives in
Sherwood Forest, Ontario, Canada.

David Nakahara started studying Tai Chi and Kung Fu in
1974 and has taught both. He has been involved in writing
about Tai Chi for many years, and produced and directed
David Carradine's Tai Chi Workout on video.

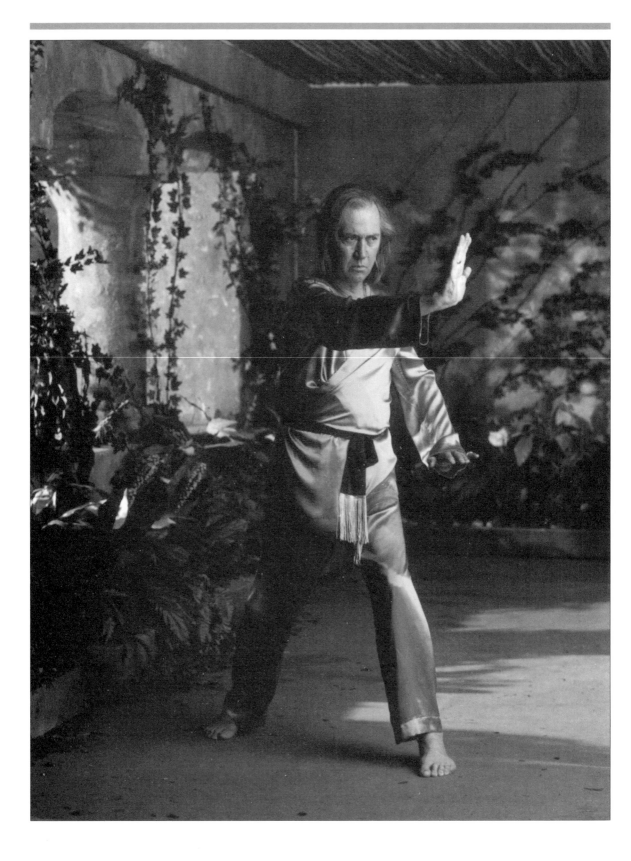

DAVID CARRADINE'S
TAI CHI
WORKOUT

David Carradine

AND

David Nakahara

TED SMART

Advice To The Reader

Before following any exercise advice on the programme contained in this book, it is recommended that you consult your doctor if you suffer from any health problems or special conditions or are in any doubt as to its suitability.

First published in Great Britain in 1994 by Boxtree Limited

Published in 1995 by The Book People Ltd.
Guardian House
Borough Road
Godalming
Surrey GU7 2AE
By arrangement with Boxtree Ltd

Concept for the book by Letticia Stafford dba I T S Entertainment

Designed by Robert Updegraff
Photography produced by Gail Jensen-Carradine and Jillian Lovink
Photographs by Mark Mainguy
Movements demonstrated by Mike Marshall and Jillian Lovink
Chinese Calligraphy by Qu Lei Lei
Origination by Adelphi Graphics

Printed and bound in Trowbridge, England by Redwood Books

A CIP catalogue entry for this book is available from the British Library.

ISBN 1 85283 475 7

CONTENTS

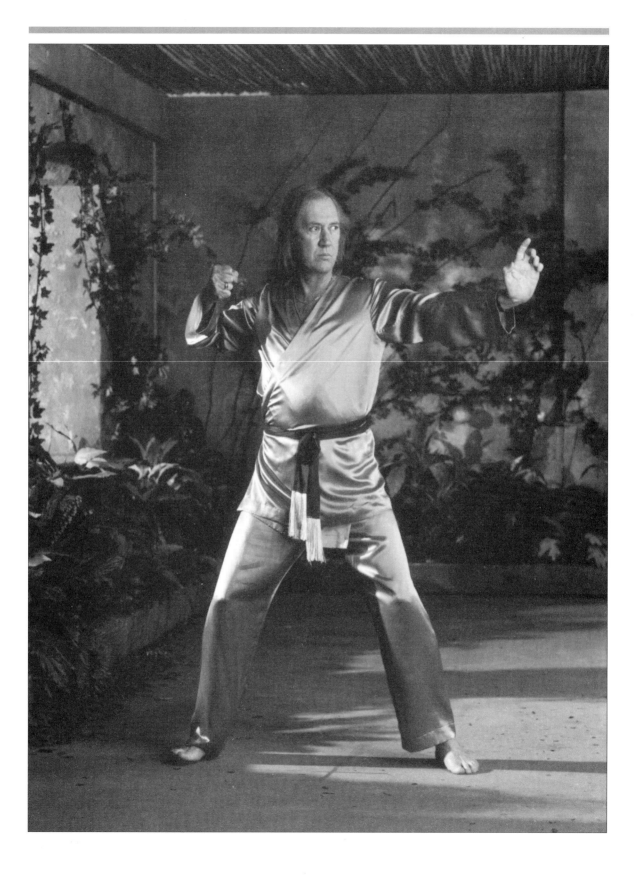

古代哲學

Tai Chi: An Ancient Philosophy

INTRODUCTION

Tai Chi is described in many different ways. Some say it is a martial art, others say it is only for health, many call it 'the art of creating energy' and some refer to it as 'meditation in motion'. Some people claim it is a physical manifestation of a philosophy called Taoism, and others describe it as a continuous flow of 'Chi Kung' or breathing exercises. It has been likened to low impact aerobics, yet others testify that it is a way of life, and even claim that it is a way to achieve spiritual enlightenment. I say it is all of these.

Tai Chi is designed to affect a person on any level one allows it to. It physically strengthens the body while encouraging flexibility and ease of movement. It is designed to increase internal energy of 'chi' flow within the body thereby increasing vitality. It will clean, relax and focus the mind, promoting creativity, sensitivity and optimism. It gives balance, emotionally, and can guide one spiritually. But the best thing about Tai Chi is that anyone can do it. You do not have to be a fine physical specimen, nor do you have to be a mental giant. You just have to have a desire to be physically and/or mentally healthy. You must value feeling good and you must believe that Tai Chi can work. Belief comes from understanding; this book will not only give you the tools to learn and practise Tai Chi, but will also try to explain the various components that make Tai Chi what it is.

> *When Tao is lost, there is goodness.*
> *When goodness is lost, there is kindness.*
> *When kindness is lost, there is justice.*
> *When justice is lost, there is ritual.*
> *Now ritual is the husk of faith and loyalty, the beginning of confusion*

THE TAO TE CHING
by Lao Tsu
600 BC

9

古代哲學

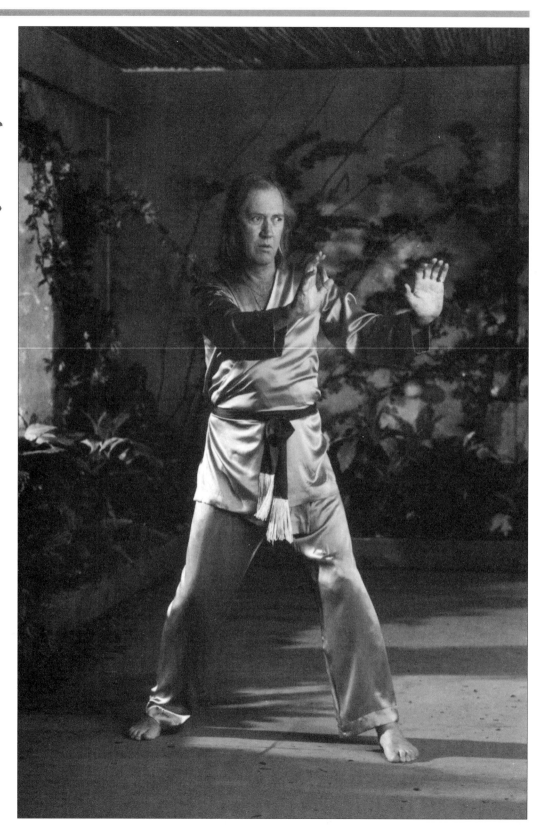

History

The ancient Chinese spent thousands of years studying, researching and developing the health and power of the human mind and body. In the beginning, their hopes were motivated by the prospect of attaining spiritual enlightenment and complete unity with the mysterious and inscrutable forces of the universe. Later, as human societies grew, man distanced himself from nature, so the works of the ancients focused on helping people maintain longevity, morality and contact with a natural life. The ancients wrote the *I Ching* (The Book of Changes) which would serve as the theoretical basis of the dynamic forces that make up the universe. The *Yellow Emperor*, a medical journal, and later the *Tao Te Ching* a philosophy manual, were also created. Even later, the old masters found a need to develop extraordinary fighting prowess to preserve their societies and social order. Thus, the Shaolin Monks organized and refined external martial arts and demonstrated incredible feats of athleticism and martial skill. Others developed internal martial arts in such styles as 'Pa Kua', 'Tai Chi' and 'Hsing-I' with which they exhibited great inner power. Through thousands of years of study and refinement, whether the field was spiritual, medical or martial, the key to human self-development was the same: in order to realize and unleash human potential and awareness, the mind, body and soul must be 'cleansed'. Whether the practitioner was a fighter, healer or sage, this cleansing was achieved through meditation, movement and inner spiritual searching. In fact, the sage was often a healer and a martial artist, the martial artist often developed into a healer and then finally a sage. This is quite unlike western philosophy where human development is kept separate. You rarely find a professional boxer becoming a doctor and then finally a priest. Even less likely would be to practise all three simultaneously. Yet this was common in old China.

Knowing ignorance is strength.
Ignoring knowledge is sickness.

If one is sick of sickness, then one is not sick.
The sage is not sick because he is sick of sickness.
Therefore he is not sick.

Lao Tsu

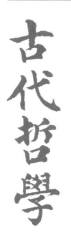

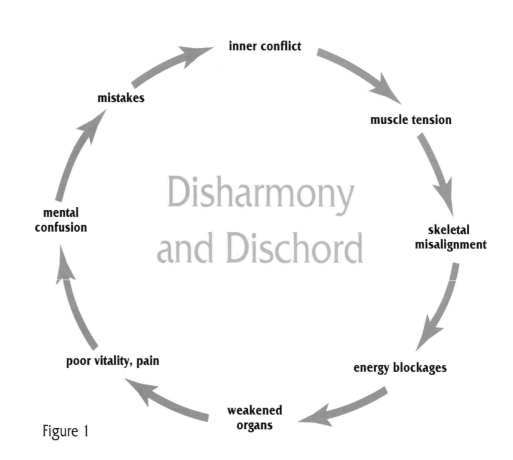

inner conflict

mistakes

muscle tension

mental
confusion

Disharmony
and Dischord

skeletal
misalignment

poor vitality, pain

energy blockages

weakened
organs

Figure 1

The West is only just beginning to adopt a holistic approach to health; by contrast, in the East a far more sophisticated understanding has developed of the relationship between mind and body, to the extent that one can even associate specific emotions with specific internal organs. The Ancients found that the internal organs, muscular flexibility and strength, skeletal alignment, skin tone, the circulatory system and metabolism were affected by ones emotional state, mental harmony and moral behaviour. For instance, inner conflict will cause muscles to tighten which forces bones to lose alignment, inhibiting energy and blood flow. This will weaken an internal organ which imbalances the entire internal system, depleting vitality and strength. This will in turn promote mental stress which leads to clouded thinking, causing misunderstandings and mistakes, and resulting in disharmony with others, leaving one with inner conflict. (See Figure 1)

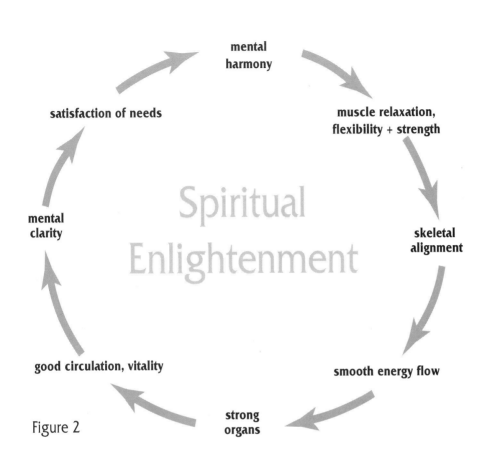

Figure 2

Conversely, mental harmony allows the muscles to relax and thus realign the skeletal system; this releases energy and boosts blood circulation, thus nourishing the internal organs and strengthening the body. This in turn increases vitality and energy, promoting clear and positive thinking which enables you to accomplish your goals. This accomplishment leads to increased self-esteem, and a feeling of being in tune with your surroundings resulting in inner peace and mental harmony. (See Figure 2)

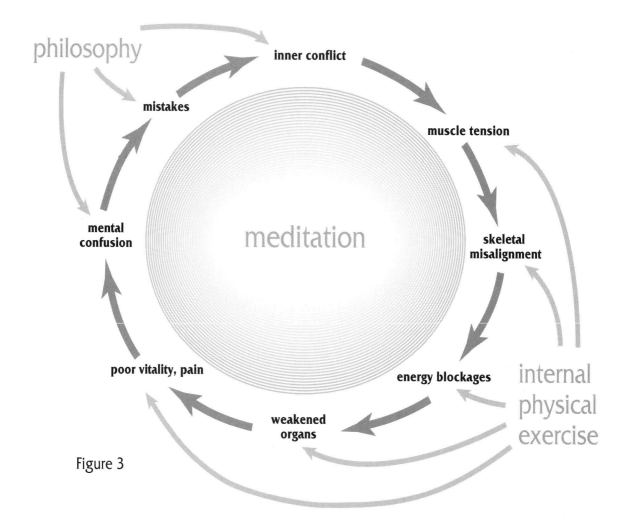

philosophy

inner conflict

mistakes

muscle tension

mental
confusion

meditation

skeletal
misalignment

poor vitality, pain

internal
physical
exercise

weakened
organs

energy blockages

Figure 3

This 'health cycle' can be maintained in a variety of ways. In Figure 3 we see that we can enter the health cycle at any point. In fact, a balanced and all-encompassing approach is more effective. Tai Chi is unique in that it embodies all the solutions shown in the chart. Tai Chi is practised in a meditative state to induce physical and mental relaxation, self-awareness and sensitivity. The moves develop flexibility, balance, strength, co-ordination, skeletal alignment, and body linkage. The slow twisting and torquing movements of the torso massage the internal organs, thereby improving their function. With the focusing of the mind combined with precise and co-ordinated movement, your natural internal energy is stimulated and spread throughout the body. Finally, the flowing and natural movement teaches the mind to 'be'. If one moves with grace and balance, one begins to live with grace and balance. Thus, Tai Chi is a way to maintain the health cycle with the multiple solutions working simultaneously.

Why does everyone like the Tao so much at first?

Isn't it because you find what you seek and are forgiven when you sin?

Therefore this is the greatest treasure of the universe.

Lao Tsu

Taoism

There are several principles and practices that constitute Taoist philosophy. Volumes of books have been written on how to apply these methods either physically, emotionally, spiritually, or philosophically. We will try to explain two central themes of Taoism. The most popular concept is 'Yin and Yang' which is also a part of many other eastern philosophies.

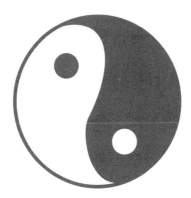

The Yin and Yang symbol is a call for balance in life: too much of anything is not good. For instance, courage taken too far leads to recklessness; too much strength becomes stubbornness; too much desire leads to obsession; too much power brings on corruption. In Tai Chi, extending too far or committing too much force leads to loss of balance. The symbol shows us that there is always a touch of black within white and white contained in black: a good man has some feminine qualities; a great lie has a semblance of truth, a good sword has some flexibility, a good leader is sometimes subservient. Tai Chi follows this principle, and is often described as 'steel within cotton'. Tai Chi is internally hard: the bones become strong and dense, the body's structure is solid. Externally, Tai Chi is soft: the muscles are relaxed, pliable and sensitive.

Another theory associated with Taoism is 'Wei Wu Wei', which loosely translates as 'do without doing, act without action'. The Taoist believes that great creativity and power would flow through all of us if we would let it. We inhibit ourselves because we try too hard, think too much and do not believe. Have you ever played a sport, played a musical

15

古代哲學

instrument or participated in a performance where you have felt as though everything was effortless and working as if you were on 'autopilot'? This state of being is what the Taoist will feel is natural, desirable, and something to work towards in everyday life.

Tao Te Ching by Lao Tsu

The poems that feature in this book are excerpts from the *Tao Te Ching*, by Lao Tsu. This ancient Chinese classic, written in the sixth century BC, has been translated more than any other book in the world with the exception of the Bible. Little is known about Lao Tsu, other than that he was the Imperial Archive Keeper. He was also once visited by Confucius who came away in awe of him. In his old age, Lao Tsu became disillusioned with society and decided to ride off into the desert. A gatekeeper recognized him and begged him to write down his teachings. He then wrote the eighty-one poems which are the *Tao Te Ching*.

Loosely and literally translated, 'Tao' means, 'the way'. 'Te' is virtue, but should not be limited to a moral context as virtue also means innate, creative human potential; 'Ching' labels the work as classic. Some refer to the Tao Te Ching as 'the art of living'. It addresses the dynamics of war, leadership, society, relationships, spiritual searching, nature and movement. It brings to life principles of naturalness, balance, duality, non-interference and other concepts associated with Taoist philosophy. Tai Chi is considered a Taoist martial art, which transforms these principles into movement, self-defence and self-cultivation. In short, one could say that Tai Chi is a physical manifestation of Taoist concepts or conversely, the *Tao Te Ching* is a philosophical interpretation of Tai Chi strategy.

Breathing and Meditation

呼吸静思

呼吸静思

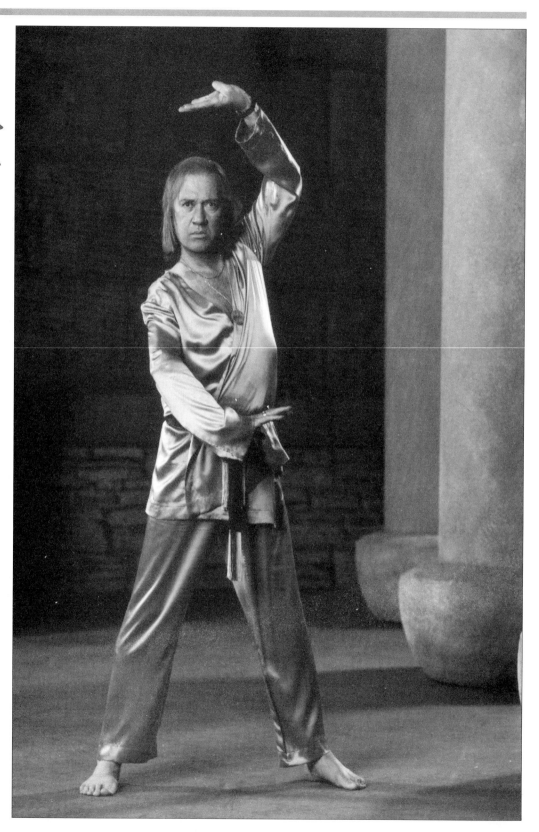

Peace is easily maintained;
Trouble is easily overcome before it starts.
The brittle is easily shattered;
The small is easily scattered.
Deal with it before it happens.
Lao Tsu

BREATHING AND MEDITATION

Chi

Accepting the existence of chi is important to having a holistic view of health. When you meditate and practise breathing you are exerting influence on your chi. Chi is energy. In both Eastern and Western philosphy, everything in the universe is made up of energy, or chi, the only difference between things being the frequency of their vibration. For instance, a solid object is energy vibrating at a low frequency, whereas fire is energy vibrating at a high frequency. The East treats everything like one big energy field, all is a connected part of a larger picture: objects, thoughts, emotions, sounds, the human body and psychic abilities are all just different forms of energy, or chi, that constantly interrelate and affect each other. For instance, certain emotions affect certain internal organs which can be healed by certain sounds, colours and thoughts. We are creatures of chi and are affected by all that is of chi. There are various types, classifications and sources of chi. There is prenatal chi, postnatal chi, heaven chi, earth chi, man chi, chi in the air, food, herbs and water. We shall be concerned with man or human chi and always refer to it simply as chi.

Chi circulates throughout the body in pathways called meridians. There are main meridians which branch off to smaller meridians. The larger meridians connect and nourish the organs of the body. The key to health is to keep this chi flowing smoothly through the meridians. Chi flow is similar to the way water flows through a system of hoses. When the muscles tighten or the bones lose alignment, these hoses, or meridians, become 'pinched'. Before long, the chi clogs up and a dam, or blockage occurs. The surrounding area of the body, or an associated internal organ becomes imbalanced and weakened. In the short term, this may lead to a minor injury; in the long term, disease may occur. The blockages can be unclogged by a healer (acupuncturist or acupressurist) or with Tai Chi. Tai Chi conditions and relaxes the muscles, releasing tension and chi blockages. The postures align the body's skeletal system, keeping the meridians clear. The joints of the body open up, easing chi circulation. Finally, by combining physical movement, imagination, sensitivity, breathing and relaxation one learns to move and circulate the chi.

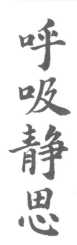

So sometimes things are ahead and sometimes they are behind;
Sometimes breathing is hard, sometimes it comes easily;
Sometimes there is strength and sometimes weakness;
Sometimes one is up and sometimes down.

Therefore the sage avoids extremes, excesses, and complacency.

Lao Tsu

Breathing

In all of the Chinese health arts, breathing is very important and can be very complex. There are some breathing techniques that are so powerful in how they affect chi flow that they can actually damage or overheat the body internally. This book will stick to very simple, safe, yet effective breathing techniques. Only do more advanced breathing under the close supervision of a qualified teacher.

Concentrate on lowering your breathing. Imagine that your lungs expand into your abdomen area - do not force this, just direct your awareness to this region. Your breathing will feel deeper, fuller and more relaxed. The longer your inhalations and exhalations, the better, but again don't force this. Deep, relaxed breathing increases blood circulation and has a profound calming affect. Have you ever noticed that when you are tense or frustrated someone will often say, 'take a deep breath'? It's good advice because it relaxes and clears the mind and body.

The average person takes about sixteen breaths (one breath is one inhalation and one exhalation) per minute. When you practise relaxed, lower breathing during meditation, it may drop to between eight and twelve breaths per minute. If you have been meditating for a while (perhaps a year), you will take about four to six breaths per minute during meditation, and about eight breaths during normal activity.

The number of breaths is proportional to how many thoughts you have during meditation. When meditating, you will find your breathing will slow as you let go of extraneous thoughts. There are those who believe that a lifetime can be measured by the number of 'thoughts' or breaths one experiences. Thus, the fewer breaths a person takes, the longer he or she will live. Whenever you practise Tai Chi, meditate, exercise, walk or whatever, lower and relax your breathing.

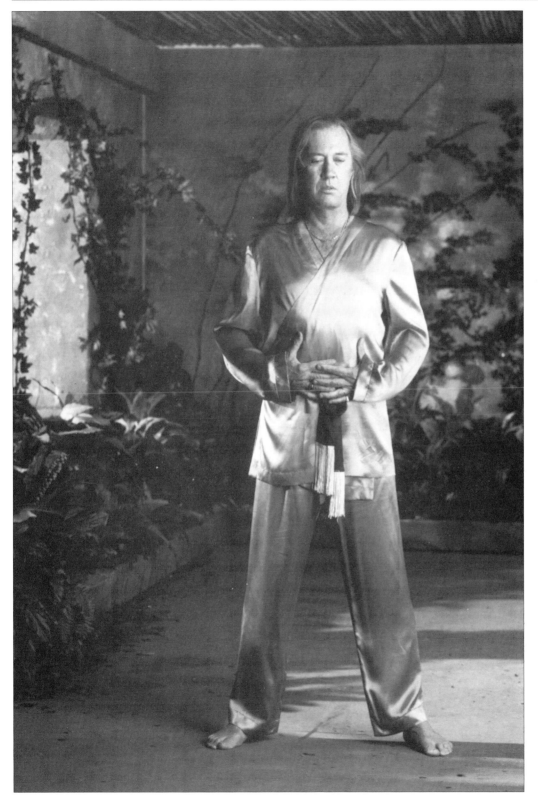

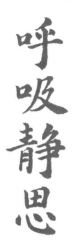

Meditation

There are several different forms and styles of meditation. There are meditations for meridian chi flow, rejuvenation of the internal organs, perception and awareness, mental and physical cleansing, focusing and developing spirit and intent; there are chi-packing meditations, chakra meditations, moving meditations, sleeping meditations, standing, sitting and lying meditations. Some meditations are quite powerful and can be harmful if done incorrectly, others are mild but safer. These meditations are effective yet safe to perform without the luxury of a teacher to monitor progress.

Wu Chi Position

The first position is called the Wu Chi position. This is actually the first posture of the Tai Chi form. This meditation is good to do before Tai Chi or prior to the other standing meditation. The purpose of this meditation is to clear the mind and relax the body.

Begin by assuming the natural standing position with feet shoulder-width apart and facing forwards, and arms hanging loosely at your sides. Knees should be slightly bent, but not locked, allowing your internal energy to flow more freely. Weight should be evenly distributed on both feet without excess pressure on the knees. The tip of the tongue should touch the roof of your mouth slightly. You should push your lower back outwards, and contract the anal sphincter. As you gaze forward imagine that your entire body is suspended from above, through the crown point at the very top of the head.

Take a deep breath down into your lower abdomen and calm your mind. Imagine a plane of light scanning down your body releasing tension. From the crown point, begin to relax the top of the head. Continue through the back and sides of the head, then down the face and jaw. Release the tightness from the entire neck area and let the relaxation pass downwards through the shoulders, upper back, chest and upper arms. Continue to take deep breaths as you feel your entire body enter a deeper state of relaxation.

Now, let go of the tension and stress in the abdomen region and lower back area and feel the release in the elbows, forearms, wrists and fingers. Continue to let the tightness melt away through the entire trunk area and upper leg region, through the knees, lower legs and finally the ankles and feet.

Breathe deeply into the lower abdomen and feel all the stress and tension from your entire body sink down and out through your feet. Relax...relax...relax....

You should practise holding this position for about three minutes. This will allow you to calm your mind and make your breathing deeper and slower-paced. With your entire body relaxed and your mind clear, you now have the ideal state in which you can practise Tai Chi or do other meditation.

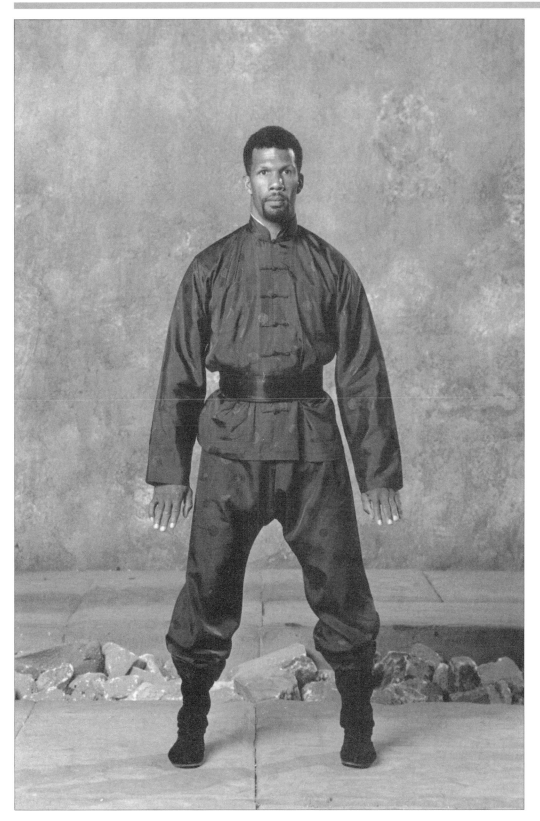

呼吸静思

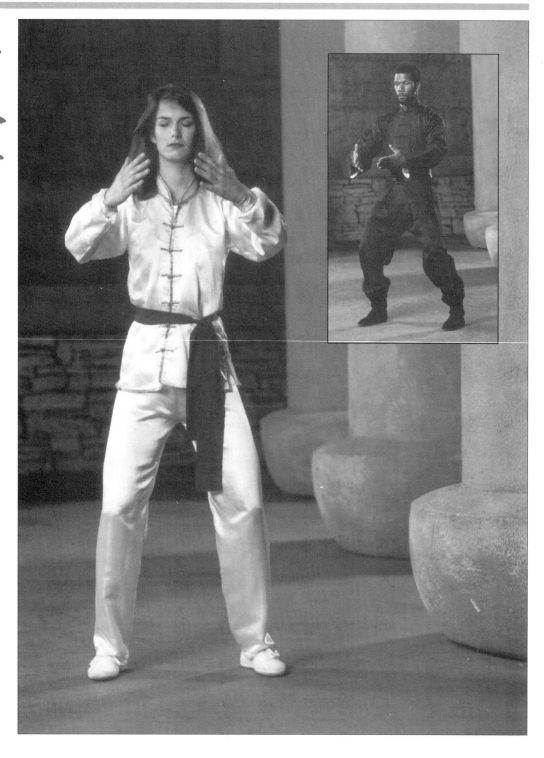

Holding The Ball

This position is good for Tai Chi practitioners and allows chi to flow to the hands. Because you are standing, the legs and back are strengthened and the chi can more easily flow through the lower body.

Begin by assuming the natural standing position with your feet shoulder-width apart and facing forward, with knees slightly bent. Arms should hang loosely at the sides and the eyes gaze forward, exactly as in the Wu Chi position. The height of the stance can vary according to your preference. As your legs strengthen, you will find that you can hold this stance lower and for a longer period of time.

Again, weight should be evenly distributed on both feet without excessive pressure on the knees. Now, make sure your spine is straight by tucking your bottom in and slightly contracting the anal sphincter. Next, raise both arms up as if holding a ball in front of your chest with palms facing the chest and fingers spread apart slightly. Round the shoulders and drop the elbows. The distance between your hands can vary from three to ten inches (7.5-25cm).

Breathe deeply into your lower abdomen as you relax into the stance and feel your body sink into your feet. Place the tongue in a curled position gently touching the roof of the mouth and slightly contract the anal sphincter. Continue to focus on your breathing, placing your awareness on the lower tan tien point. This point is located about one and a half inches below the navel and a third of the way back in the body. This is considered the first major energy centre. Imagine your whole body is suspended from the crown point of the head as if you were a puppet hanging from a string.

Hold this standing position for at least five minutes. At first it will feel uncomfortable, and your shoulders and arms will feel tense and ache. If your arms do tire, then assume the lower hand position. Simply lower your arms so that the palms are now pointing toward the lower tan tien. Hold this position for at least five minutes and then return to the upper position for five minutes. Try to meditate up to thirty minutes per session but at least do it for five minutes daily.

Remember to start out with the Wu Chi position. You may either use the upper or lower position or alternate. Meditate either before your workout, after your workout, or instead of your workout.

25

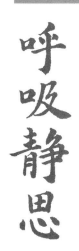

The five colours blind the eye.
The five tones deafen the ear.
The five flavours dull the taste.
Racing and hunting madden the mind.
Precious things lead one astray.

Therefore the sage is guided by what he feels and not by what he sees.
He lets go of that and chooses this.
Lao Tsu

Physical Sensations During Meditation

Meditation will cause you to experience many new sensations because you are stimulating chi flow and you are increasing awareness of your internal body. You will probably feel most of the feelings listed in the chart. The aching sensations are usually a result of incorrect posture and the muscles lacking endurance. Your body will develop with practise and eventually you will be able to hold your posture with no discomfort. This may take a few months. You may also experience other sensations not listed. Everyone is unique.

SENSATIONS DURING MEDITATION

Negative Sensations

Aching shoulders	Normal at first, but make sure your shoulders are relaxed and drooping.
Aching neck	This means you could be suffering from mental tension; check the tension in your jaw. Do neck rolls and self massage and meditate in the Wu Chi position .
Aching knees	Check that your weight is distributed evenly and make sure that your knees are not bent further forward than your toes.
Aching back	Check your posture. Make sure your bottom is not sticking out.
Aching arms	Normal at first but do extra arm swings as part of your programme.
Aching feet	Normal at first but during meditation shift your feet to find a comfortable position.
Aching head	Direct your awareness towards your feet. Practise self massage to your head and neck, and make sure your tongue touches roof of your mouth.
Bloated stomach	This is sometimes a sign that your breathing is too forced. Check your diet and massage your stomach.

Positive Sensations

Sweating	Normal. A sign that the body is cleansing itself.
Numbness	Normal. A sign that chi is flowing.
Tingling	Normal. A sign that chi is flowing.
Body Heat	Normal. A sign that chi is flowing. When energy flows it heats the body.
Trembling	Normal. A sign that chi is flowing.
Feeling Asymmetrical	Normal. The body is trying to rebalance itself.
Yawning	A sign that you are able to relax but perhaps you are too tired.
Burping	A good sign. The body is discharging toxins.
Flatulence	A good sign. The body is discharging toxins.
Diminishing or No Sensation	This may happen after practising meditation for a while. This is a sign that the meridian pathways have opened up.
Aching Old Injuries	Mostly a good sign, it means you are progressing but can sometimes mean that you are pushing yourself too hard.

太極計划

The Tai Chi Programme

太極計划

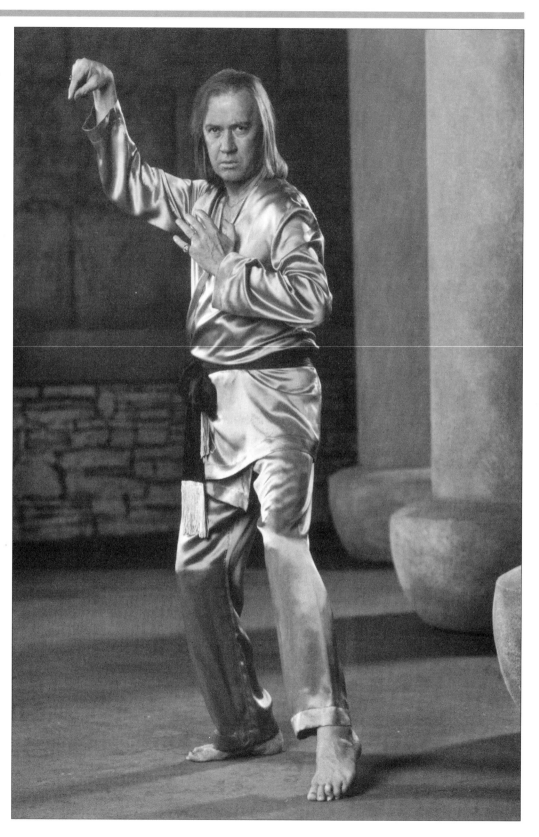

THE TAI CHI PROGRAMME

Thirteen-Week Programme

Tai Chi is best learned in stages. The components must first be learned individually, and then combined to form a complete Tai Chi form. This thirteen-week programme is in four teaching sections. The first section is Stance training, which develops the legs and footwork. The second is Chi Kung, which teaches co-ordination of the breathing and relaxation, with movement. The third section explains the individual moves of Tai Chi. These are more complicated moves that combine the stances with the upper body movements. They are isolated and repeated several times. Finally, in the fourth section, the individual movements are combined in a continuous motion creating a complete Tai Chi form.

Meditation should also be part of your programme, as it is a good supplementary training for Tai Chi.

You should practise every day! If you are busy then only do five minutes but think in terms of 'daily' not in terms of how many times per week.

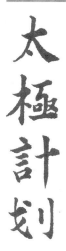

THE THIRTEEN-WEEK PROGRAMME

Weeks One to Two
Five to twenty minutes daily

The Stances
You should do the whole programme of stances in each session, gradually holding them for longer. You are aiming to be able to get into and out of each stance with ease. Your leg muscles should become strong enough to hold each posture for one minute or more.

Weeks Three to Four
Ten to twenty minutes daily

Chi Kung
Learn two new exercises every day. This is good for conditioning the upper body - the torso, the arms, the neck and back.
Also practise your stances for five to ten minutes.

Weeks Five to Eight
Ten to thirty minutes daily

Individual Tai Chi Moves
Learn each move one at a time and add one new move every day. You should spend five to ten minutes on a new move and one to two minutes practising each old move. Also practise Chi Kung for five to ten minutes and The Stances for five to ten minutes reducing the time as you learn more Tai Chi moves.

Weeks Nine to Twelve
Ten to thirty minutes daily

The Continuing Tai Chi Form
You should now be familiar with the individual moves but you need to make the transitions. Link a new move to the last old move everyday using the transitional movements. You should still practise the individual moves that you have not yet combined, for ten to twenty minutes. Also practise The Stances for five to ten minutes and Chi Kung for five to ten minutes, reducing the time the more of the combined form you learn.

Week Thirteen and onwards
Ten to thirty minutes daily

You should now have memorized the complete form but you should continue to study the exact Tai Chi postures. Practise your complete form for ten to twenty minutes, and Chi Kung for five to twenty minutes. Performing the individual Tai Chi moves and The Stances are now optional.

Training tips

The key to learning Tai Chi is steady, slow, patient progress: you cannot learn too slowly, but you can learn too quickly. It is as if you are building a house. If you do not take time to work on the basics then you will not have a good base of structure to build on. If the foundation is weak then everything built on top of the foundation will be unstable. Nothing will feel right. Remember, while you familiarize yourself physically and mentally with the exercises, you are developing strength, flexibility, and concentration. It's not as if you are not benefiting until you complete the whole form. With each section and even with each move, you have to pass through three levels of performance before moving on.

1 You must have the movement memorized and co-ordinated so that you do not have to refer to the book.

2 Your muscles have memory. The body must be able to 'pattern' the move. You must be able to do the move in the same way over and over again.

3 You must be able to do the move without tension. This is when you will gain the true benefit of the exercise. When you no longer have the constraints of unfamiliarity you will be able to feel the muscles stretching and contracting, the weight shifting, the energy flowing, the bones settling and aligning. You become one with the move or posture.

There are other things to consider for more effective training.

1 Training in the early morning is always best although any time is good.

2 Fresh, clean air is desirable.

3 Don't train in areas with a strong draught.

4 Always wear loose, comfortable clothing.

5 Wear light, thin, soft-soled shoes so that you can feel the ground.

6 Use your time economically. It is better to have shorter, concise, focused and frequent workouts rather than too long, laborious and intermittent workouts.

7 Smooth, relaxing music makes training more enjoyable.

8 Try not to eat just before or after your workout.

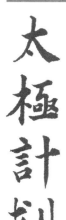

THE STANCES

This routine is great for concentrated Chi development. The postures allow you to pay particular attention to your body alignment. To have power in Tai Chi movement, you must have a good, strong and stable stance. The exercises will help develop power in your legs and you will begin to feel the relationship between the chi and the muscles.

Loosen up with the knee rotations. Begin by performing high stances, then slowly relax into them, getting deeper and lower as you gradually warm yourself up.

Try to hold each stance for one to two minutes on each side. As you progress, try to hold the stances for as long as possible.

At the end of your session, do knee rotations as a cool-down.

Be careful and wary of any knee pain. If the knees do become sore, stop and check to see if the knees are directly above the toes as they should be. Then do some knee rotations and stop for the day.

If you have very little time, just do the Horse Stance for five minutes.

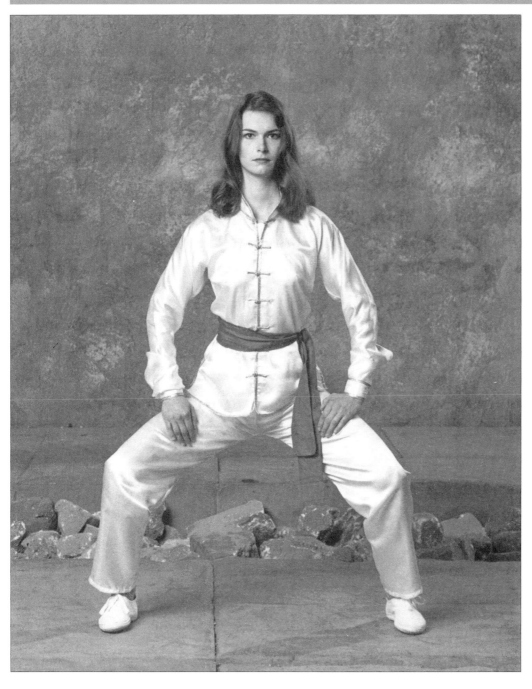

Horse Stance

Stand with your legs apart, feet parallel and facing forwards. Hold your arms naturally by your side. Your weight should be distributed evenly. Bend your knees, pushing them out to the side slightly so that the knee is above the toes. Keep the lower back pushed in and relax into the stance. Let gravity 'pull' you into the ground. Keep your back straight.

太極計划

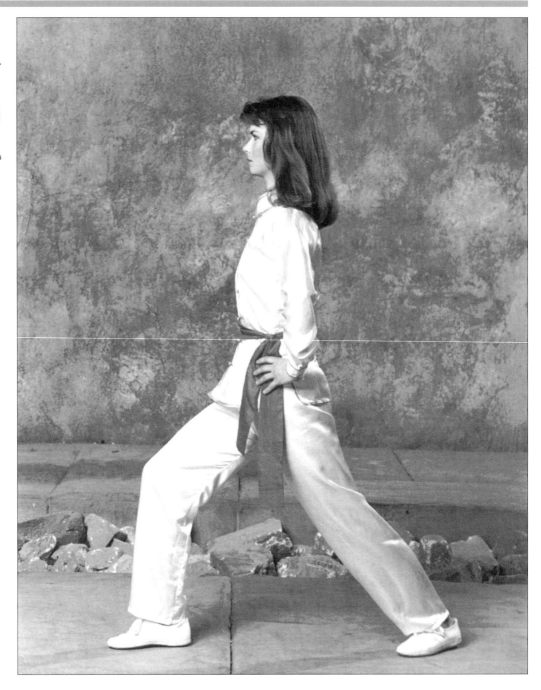

Forward Stance

Start with your right foot forward. The feet should be parallel and turned towards the left at a 45° angle. If you were to draw a line from your front foot, through the middle of your body towards the back foot the front toe would be directly in line with the back heel. Your hips should face forward.

Bend your right knee so that your lower leg is perpendicular to the floor. The left leg should be straight, outstretched at the back but keeping the knee unlocked. Your weight should be distributed equally over both legs. Breathe deeply and evenly. Feel the calf muscle stretch. By keeping the hips forward you will stretch your torso. Now switch to the left side and repeat.

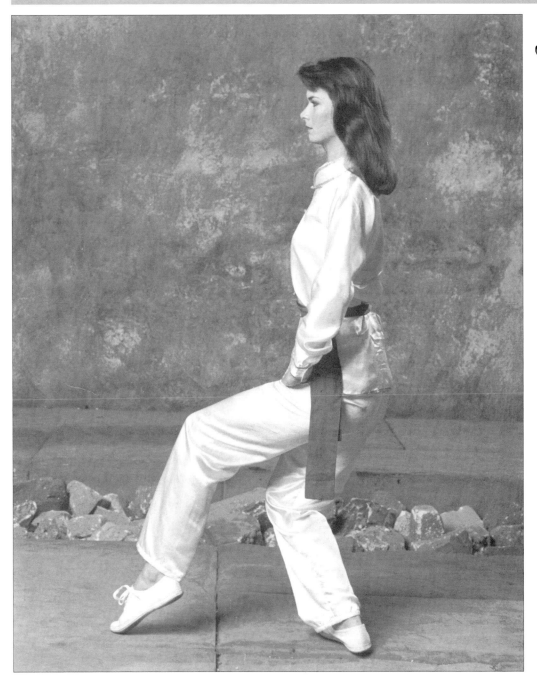

Cat Stance

Start with your left foot forward. The feet should be parallel with the toes turned towards the right at a 45° angle. Shift 80% of your weight to your back foot, lift up the left heel at the front and bend the right knee.

Drawing the same line as in Forward Stance, the front toe should line up with the back heel. Let your weight drop over the back hip, keeping both hips facing forward.

Switch to the right side and repeat.

37

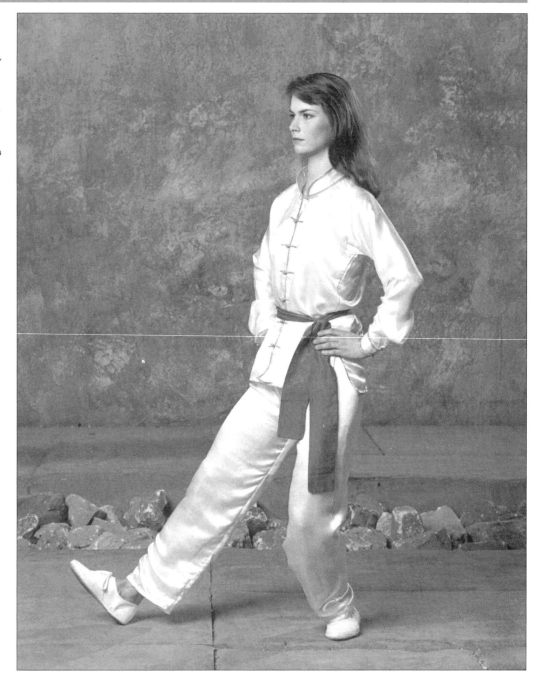

太極計划

Heel Stance

This stance is similar to the cat stance.

Start with your right foot forward. The feet should be parallel and turned towards the left at a 45° angle. Straighten but do not lock your right leg in front, bending the knee of the left leg. The heel should touch the floor with the toe pointing upwards. The heels of both feet should be in line, with 70% of your weight on the left leg at the back. Your hips should be turned about 45° towards the left. Again let the weight of your body be supported by the hip of the back leg. The higher you lift the front toe, the more you will stretch the calf muscle.

Now switch to the left and repeat.

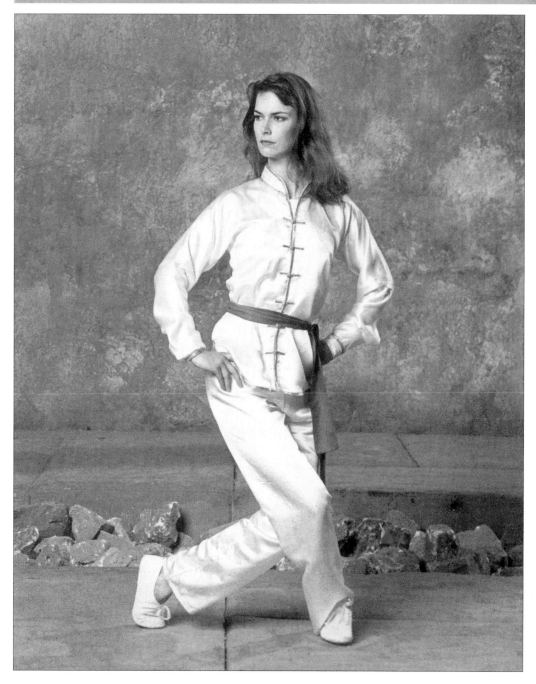

Cross Stance

Start with your right foot forward. Cross your right foot in front of the left foot. Turn your right foot 90° towards the right with your left foot, behind, directly in line with your right heel, and your weight on the ball of your foot. Your left knee should touch the back of your right knee, with your hips turned to the right slightly. Let your weight drop straight down through your hips.

Now switch to the left and repeat the stance.

太極計划

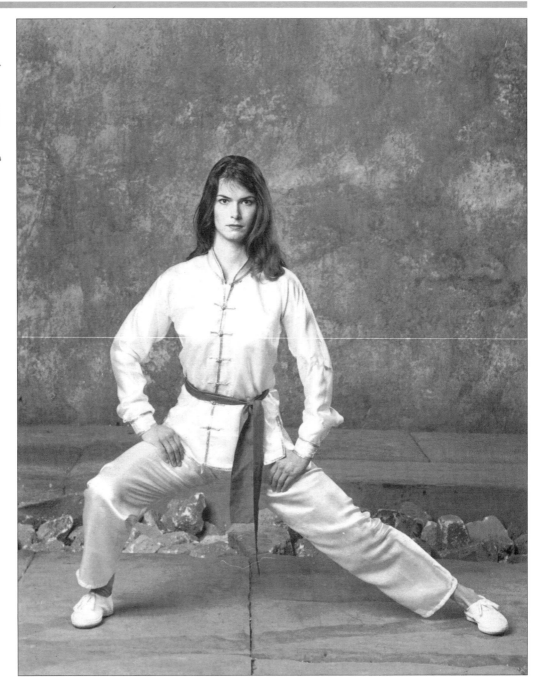

Polk Stance

Start in a horse stance. Shift your weight onto your right leg, and bend your knee. Stretch your left leg out to your side, keeping it straight. Your feet should be parallel, and pointing forwards. Try to keep the knee directly above your toes. Feel your groin stretching. Do not force yourself to lower your stance, let it happen naturally. Remember to keep your back as straight as possible, these stances work best when done in a relaxed manner, with no straining.

Now switch to the left and repeat.

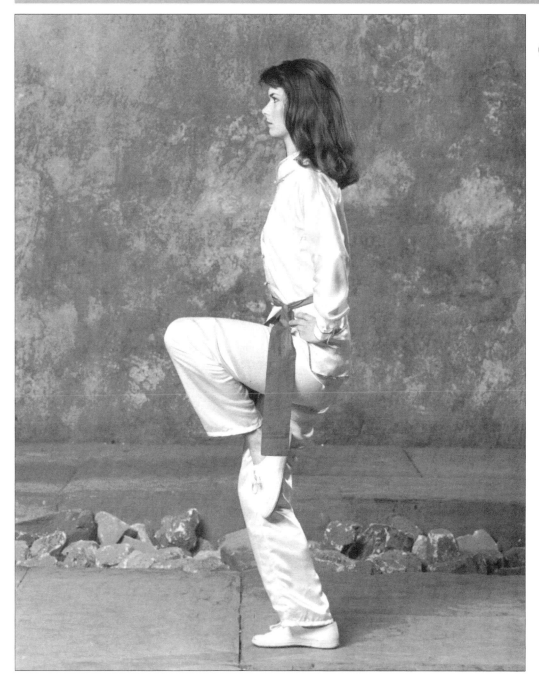

Crane Stance

Stand facing forwards, with your feet together. Lift your left knee up to be level with your hips and bend your right knee. Pull your left foot towards the inside of your right knee, point your toe toward the floor, and hold the stance.

The higher the knee the more effective the stance for strengthening the buttocks and hips. Push out the lower back to help your balance.

Now switch to the right leg and repeat.

太極計劃

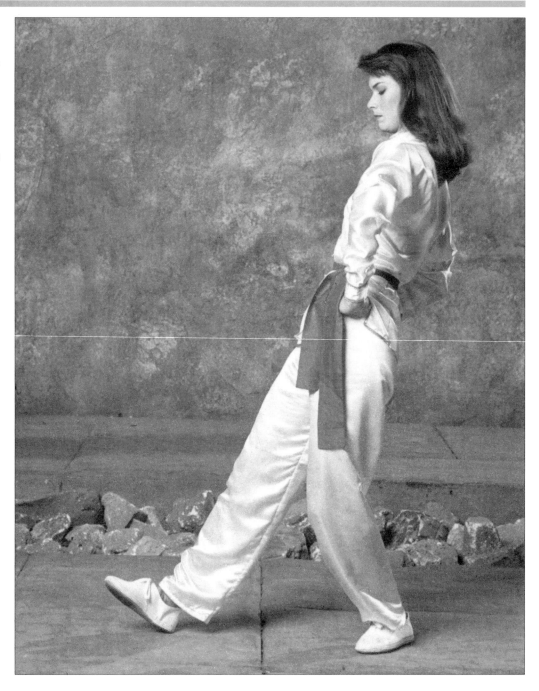

Heel Stance Back Stretch

Start from Right Heel Stance. Bending forwards from the
waist rotate your torso in large circles, clockwise and then
anticlockwise.

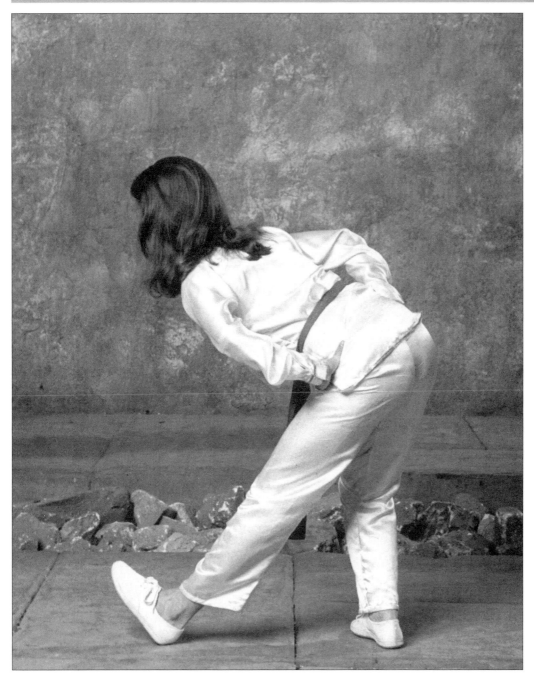

Be careful with this stretch. Move slowly and feel your back, stomach and sides stretch. A strong and healthy back is the key to health. Just about every type of movement involves the back.

Now switch to the left leg and repeat.

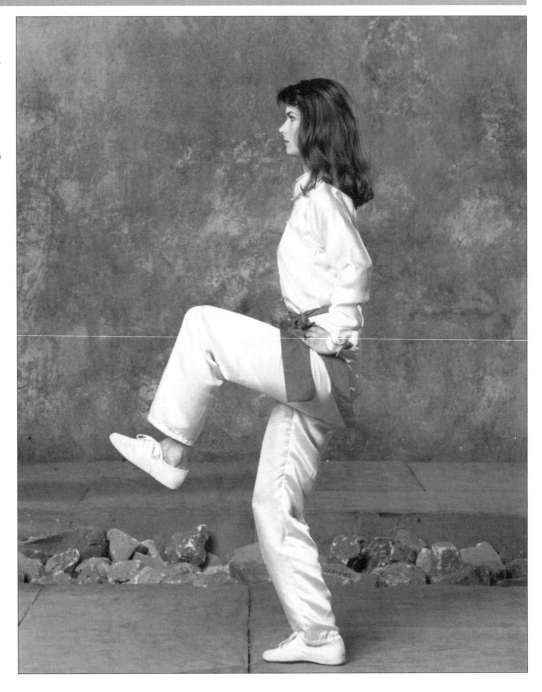

Foot Rotations

Start in a left crane stance. Rotate your left leg using the knee as a pivot point, keeping the leg hanging downwards and the bottom of your foot pointing towards the floor. Do clockwise and anticlockwise rotations. Keep the knee as stationary as possible. The larger the circle you make with the foot, the better.

Now switch to rotate the right leg.

A man is born gentle and weak.

At his death he is hard and stiff.

Green plants are tender and filled with sap.

At death they are withered and dry.

Therefore the stiff and unbending is the disciple of death.

The gentle and yielding is the disciple of life.

Lao Tsu

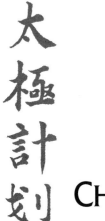

CHI KUNG

Chi Kung was invented thousands of years ago and is a predecessor of Tai Chi. These exercises are designed to increase one's energy flow and strengthen the entire body. Chi Kung literally means vital energy training. These are considered supplementary exercises and not part of the Tai Chi form but they are much easier to learn than Tai Chi. They require less knowledge, dexterity, co-ordination and practise to perform correctly. One can almost immediately enjoy the full benefits of the exercises because the moves are relatively simple. But do not underestimate the benefits of these exercises. They will help prepare your body and mind for the full Tai Chi form.

Simple can be better.

Do each movement at least eight times on both sides of the body or in both directions. Learn two new exercises each time. When learning a new exercise, do it twenty times or more. It is highly recommended to do the first five exercises every day even if you are pressed for time.

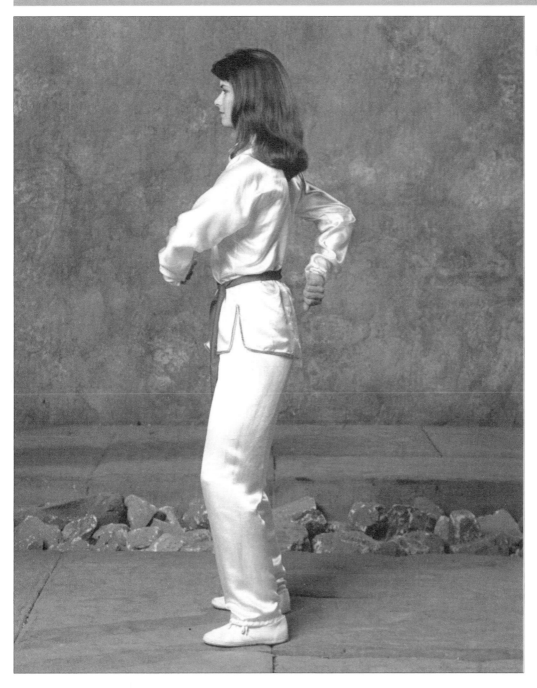

Knocking at the Gate of Life

Stand with your feet shoulder-width apart, parallel and facing forwards. Make fists with both your hands and swing your arms out to the side and back in so that the inside of your left fist hits the tan tien point and the inside of your right fist hits the lower back at the same time. Alternate and let your arms swing freely.

This exercise is good for stimulating chi flow at the main energy centres. Relax.

47

太極計划

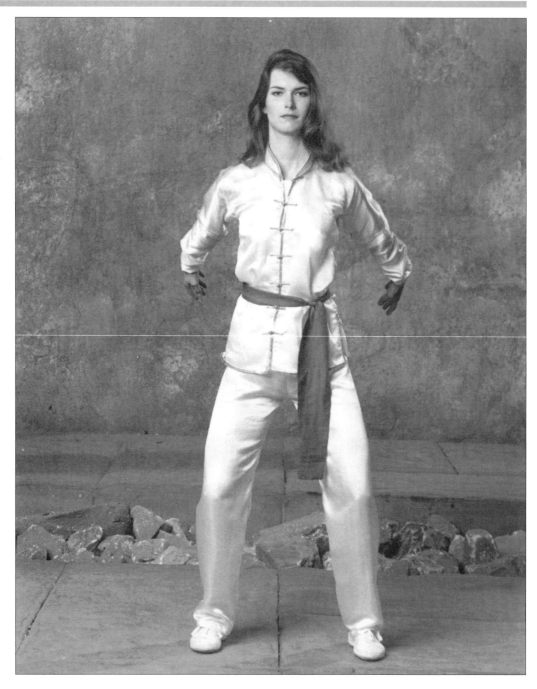

Arm Swings

Stand comfortably with your feet shoulder-width or more
apart, feet parallel and pointing forwards. Let your arms
swing forward and back, keeping them parallel and
shoulder-width apart with your palms facing one another.

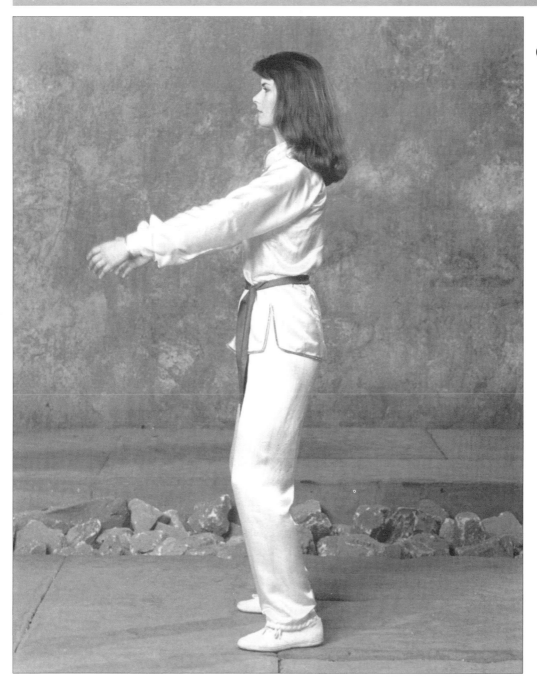

Relax your arms and shoulders. Keep the lower back pushed out. Feel your neck and shoulders relax more with each swing. Feel the energy flow to the hands.

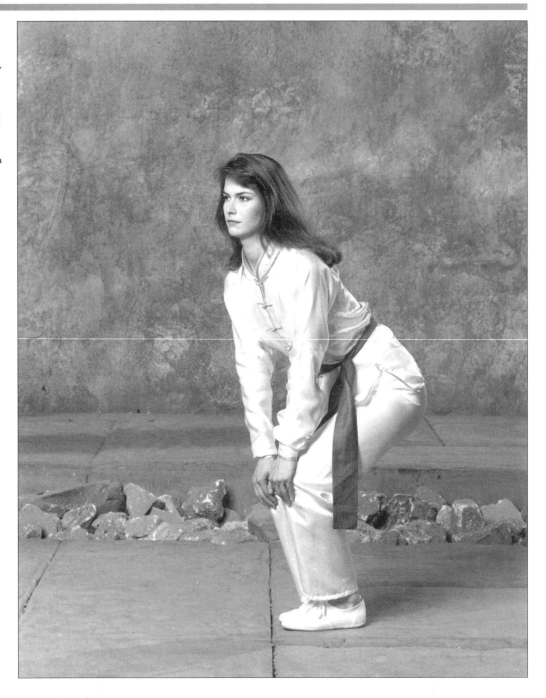

太極計划

Knee Rotations

Stand with your feet together and facing forwards. Bend over at the waist and put your hands on your knees. Bend your knees and rotate them clockwise and then anticlockwise, keeping them together. Allow your body to move naturally with the rotations.

Be careful. If your knees hurt then either stop the move or bend less. This exercise will strengthen the ligaments, tendons and cartilage of the knee. This movement will also enhance your ability to maintain balance and stability.

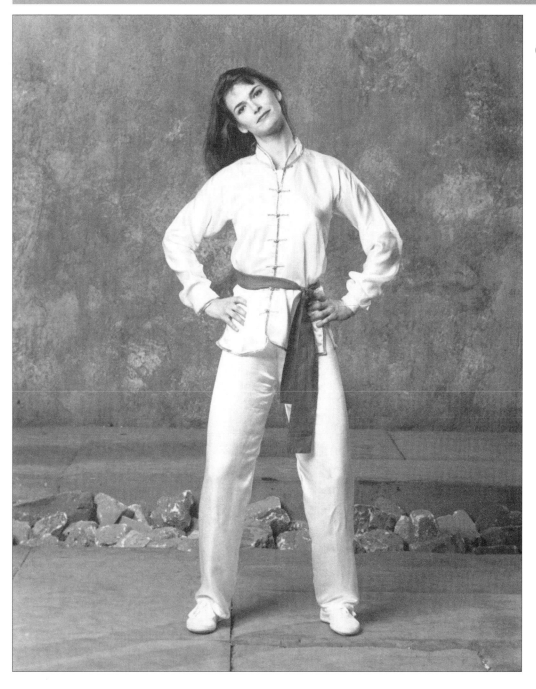

Head Rotations

Stand comfortably with your feet apart, and arms naturally by your side. Raise your chin to stretch your neck. Then make a circle moving your head up and down, rotating it clockwise and then anticlockwise. Let the stretch relieve tension in your neck. Stress can cause the body to tire and age. Let the mental tension leave your body, let the negative thoughts go and replace them with pleasant thoughts.

太極計划

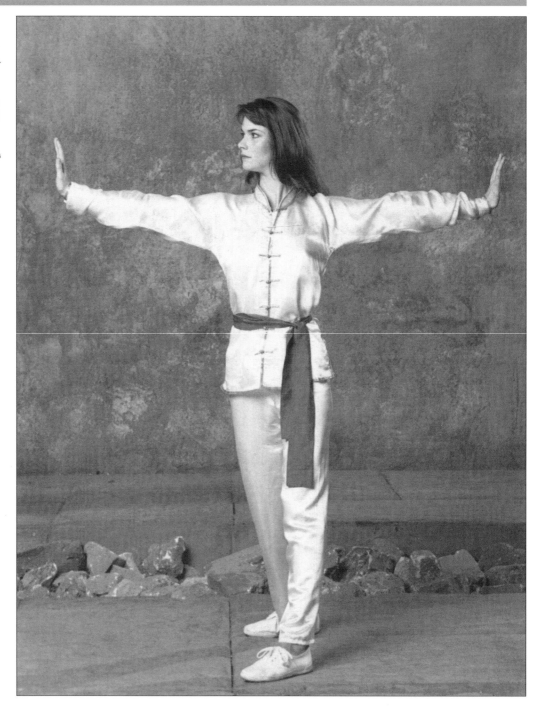

Chi Kung Front/Back Stretch

Stand with your feet shoulder-width apart, parallel and facing forwards. Extend your left arm in front of your body, and your right arm to the back. Keep your fingers pointing upwards, and palms facing away from your body. Now, turning, push your right arm out in front and your left hand behind. Allow your arms to bend as you turn, and your torso to rotate with the move. Feel your torso torque as you do this. Always exhale as you extend your arms, and inhale as you bring them into your body.

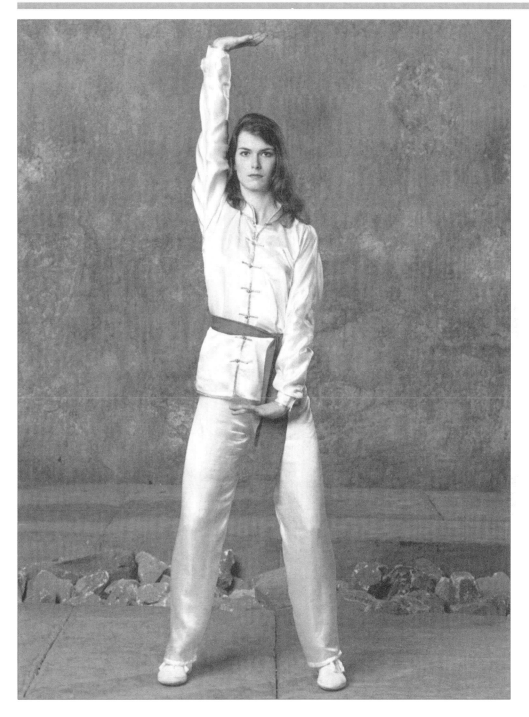

Hi-Low Stretch

Stand with your feet shoulder-width apart, parallel and facing forwards. Extend your right arm up above your head, keeping it straight, with your palm facing upwards; extend your left arm down beside your body, keeping the arm straight, with your palm facing down.

Relax and stretch as if you are waking from a nap. Now, swap: bend your arms, and allow them to cross in front of your body as you extend your left arm up above, and your right arm down. Continue to switch back and forth.

Feel your shoulders, arms and back stretching.

53

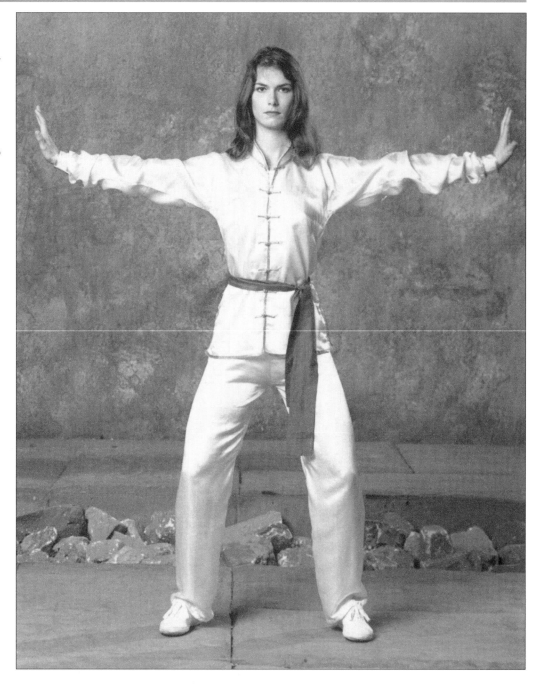

太極計划

Chi Kung Side Stretch

Stand with your feet shoulder-width apart, parallel and pointing forwards. Pull your hands up to the centre of your chest, holding them just in front, with palms facing in. Push both hands out to either side, palms facing out, straightening the arms. Then bend your arms at the elbows to bring your hands in, keeping the palms facing outwards. Keep pushing out to your sides, exhaling as you push out and inhale as you pull in. Keep your fingers pulled back, perpendicular to your arms, throughout.

Feel the energy in the fingers. This exercise will tone and strengthen your upper body. Breathe deeply and evenly.

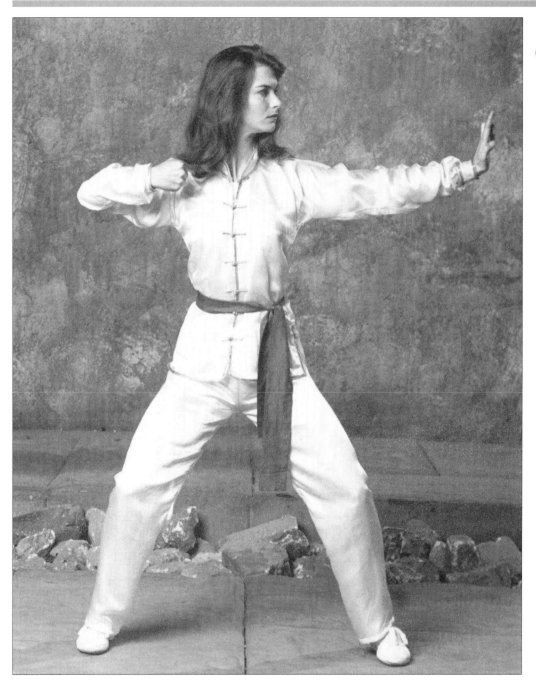

Drawing the Bow

Stand in a horse stance. Start with the left arm stretched forward with the palm facing forward and your index finger straight and facing upwards. Pull the hand back perpendicular to the arm to stretch the wrist. Your right hand clenches a fist. Pull your right fist from the left hand back toward your armpit as if you were drawing the string of a bow. Now cross your hands, turn to the left and 'draw the bow' to the opposite side.

55

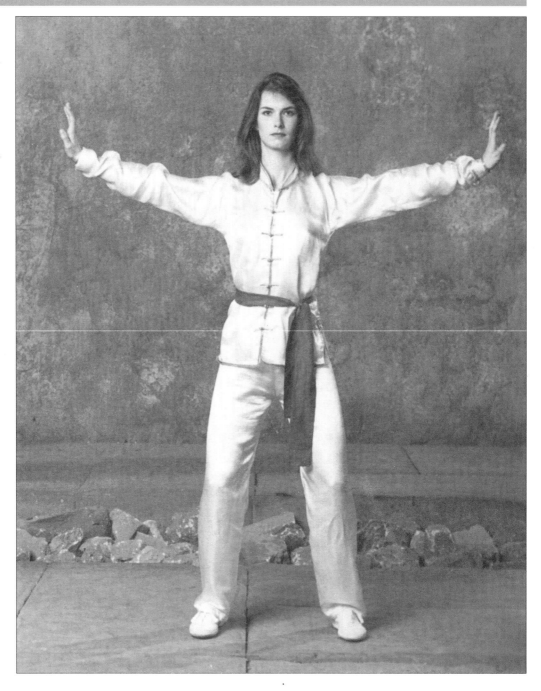

太極計划

Side Arm Rotations

Your feet should be shoulder-width apart, parallel and pointing forward. Let your arms fall naturally to your sides. Push your arms out to either side without locking the joints and pull back your fingers so that your palms face outwards. Rotate your arms backwards and then forwards keeping your arms straight and your palms facing outwards.

Feel the energy travelling through your shoulder joints, your arms and into your fingers.

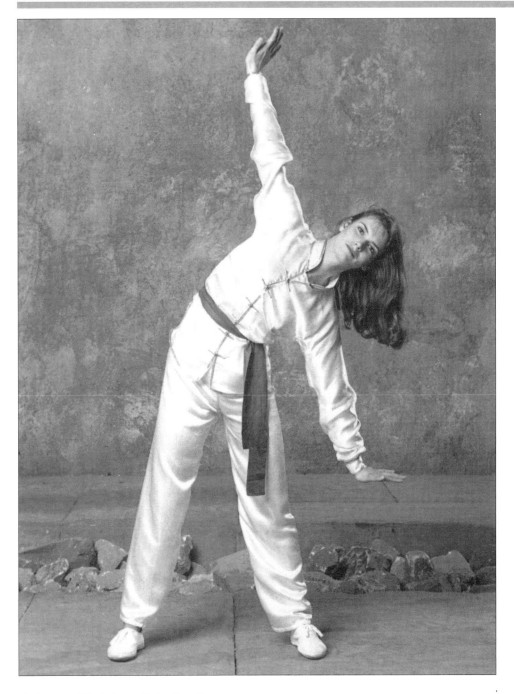

Chi Kung High Low Side Bend

Stand with your feet shoulder-width apart, parallel and pointing forwards. Start with your hands crossed in front of your chest. Bend to the left and extend your right arm upwards, and your left arm down. Keep your fingers straight and your palms facing outwards. Relax your arms in and bend them at the elbow, then push out again.

Inhale as you relax the arms and exhale as you extend out. Do eight repetitions before you switch to the other side. Make sure you keep your joints unlocked.

This exercise will stretch your side muscles while strengthening your arms. Feel the energy in your hands and fingers.

57

太極計划

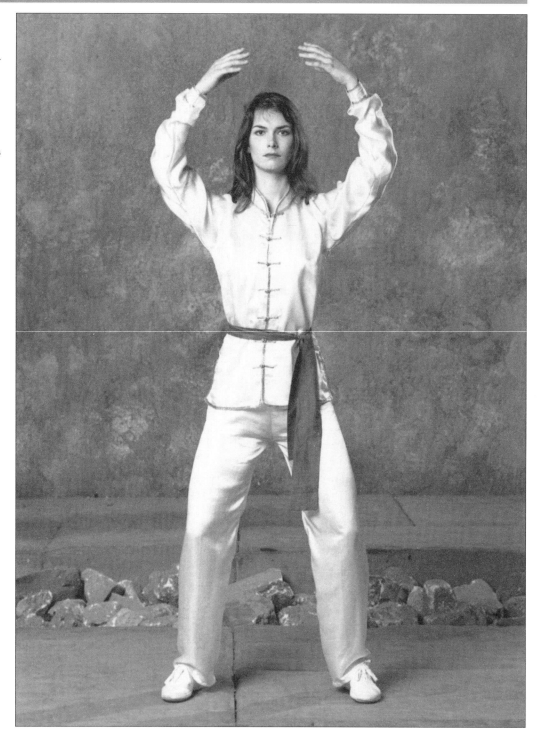

Chi Kung Downward Stretch

Stand with your feet shoulder-width apart, feet parallel and pointing forwards, and your arms resting naturally by your sides. Raise both arms in front of your face to just above your head then push both hands downwards in front of your body.

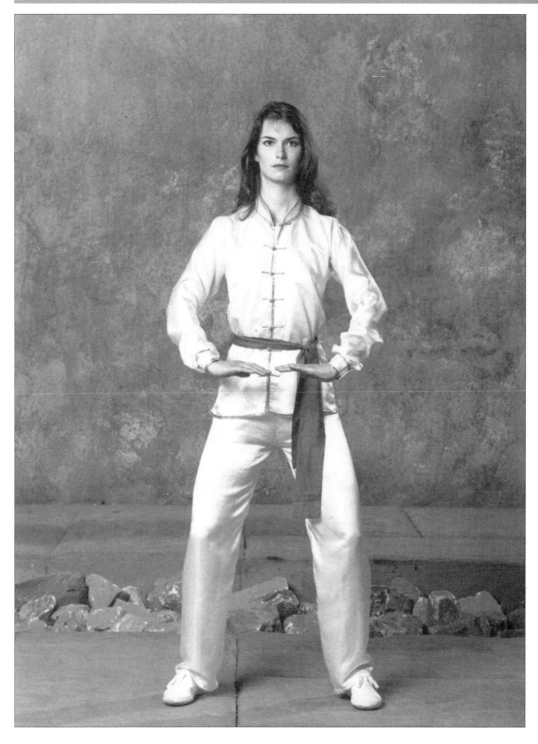

Your hands should travel in a circular motion. Exhale as you circle down, and inhale as you circle up.

Concentrate on energy circulating throughout your body, expanding in your hands. Your body must relax in order for the chi to flow properly.

59

太極計划

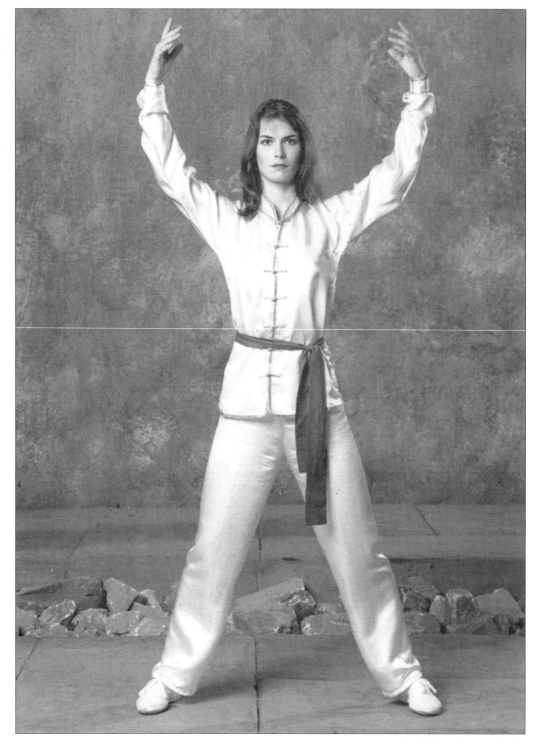

Arm Circles - Low Horse Stance

Stand in a high horse stance. Circle your arms out and upwards as if you were holding a large balloon over your head. Now let your arms swing and drop down your body, passing your knees. As your arms descend, lower your stance by bending your knees further. Smooth out

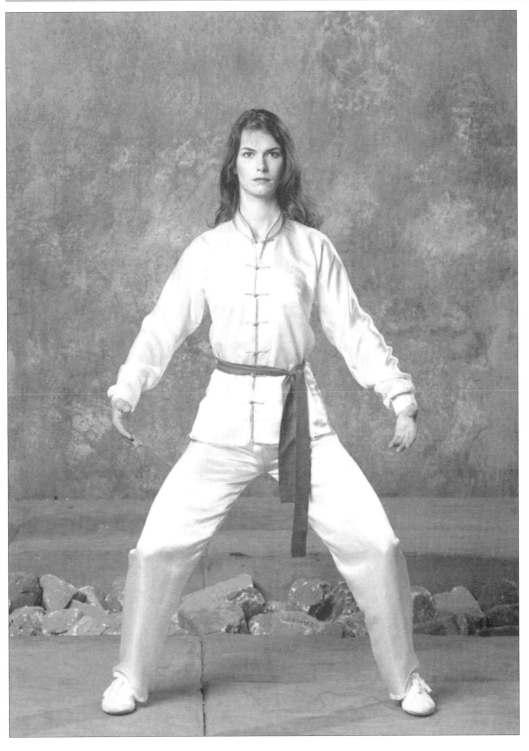

the motion so that there are no stops. Inhale as you stand
erect and exhale as you drop down. Relax and get into a
rhythm.

61

太極計划

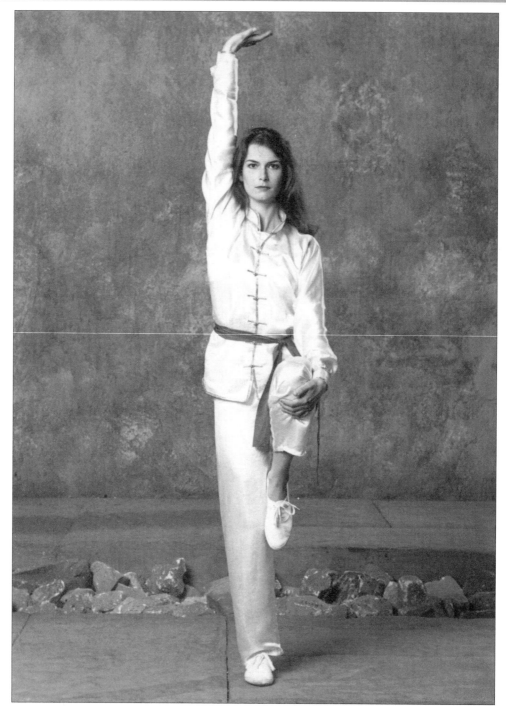

Crane Balance

Start with your feet together pointing forwards. Lift your left knee up and pull it into your chest with your left hand and raise your right hand overhead for balance, fingers stretched back and your palm facing upwards. Relax.

Push out your lower back for more balance. Hold, and then switch to the right side and repeat.

Feel the energy that is sent to your hands. Relax and concentrate. A relaxed state is the way to achieve the maximum benefits from this programme.

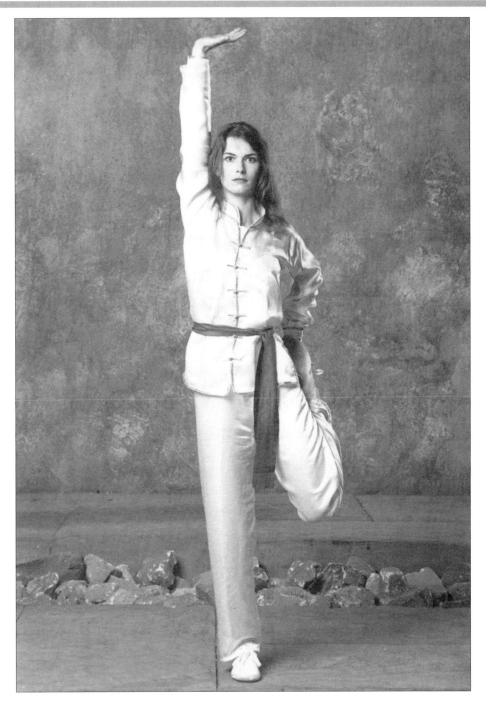

Back Crane Balance

Start with your feet together, pointing forwards. Lift your left knee, only this time move it behind you, grabbing it with your left hand and arch your back. Raise your right hand for balance, stretching back the fingers, and keeping the palm facing outwards to achieve full side stretching.

Relax your left foot for additional equilibrium. Remember to relax, lift your foot up behind you as far as possible arching your back. Now switch to the right side and repeat. Feel the thigh muscle being stretched but stop and rest if you feel strain. This exercise also works on the shoulders, arms, and lower back.

63

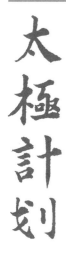

The space between heaven and earth is like a bellows.
The shape changes but not the form;
The more it moves, the more it yields.
More words count less.
Hold fast to the centre.

Lao Tsu

INDIVIDUAL TAI CHI MOVEMENTS

The best way to develop precise, quality movement in Tai Chi is to concentrate on just one move at a time. Many people learn too many moves in a short time and never get a feel for the balance and leverage, and a full practical sense of the move. By learning one move at a time your mind will not be encumbered. Your full concentration can be on developing the quality of that move, and on feeling how the chi circulates in accordance with body movement.

Do the move you are learning twenty times and practise each previously learned move eight times. If you have less time, then do familiar moves four times and unsure moves six times. Do not move on from this section until every move is memorized and your muscles have 'patterned' each movement habitually.

Once you can do the complete form it is not necessary to practise this section. You will find later that some areas of the form are weaker than others and then you may want to refer back to this section.

太極計划

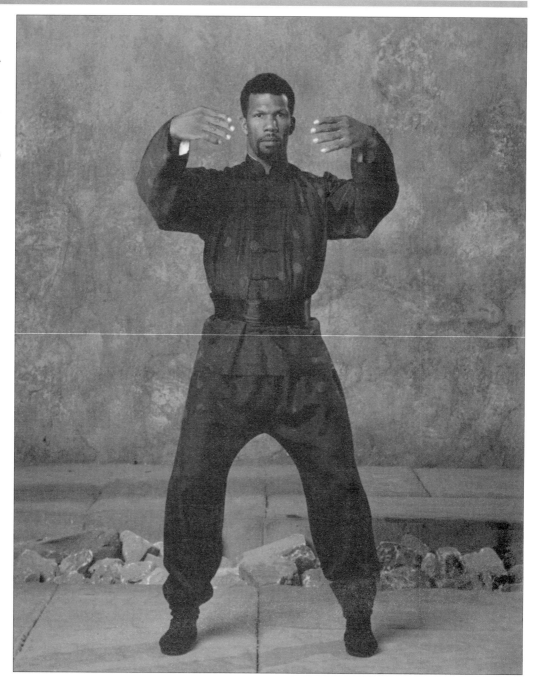

Opening Move

Stand with your feet shoulder-width apart, parallel and pointing forwards. Let your hands rest naturally at your sides. Let your elbows and shoulders drop and raise your hands up to shoulder height with your palms facing your body and the fingers of each hand pointing towards one

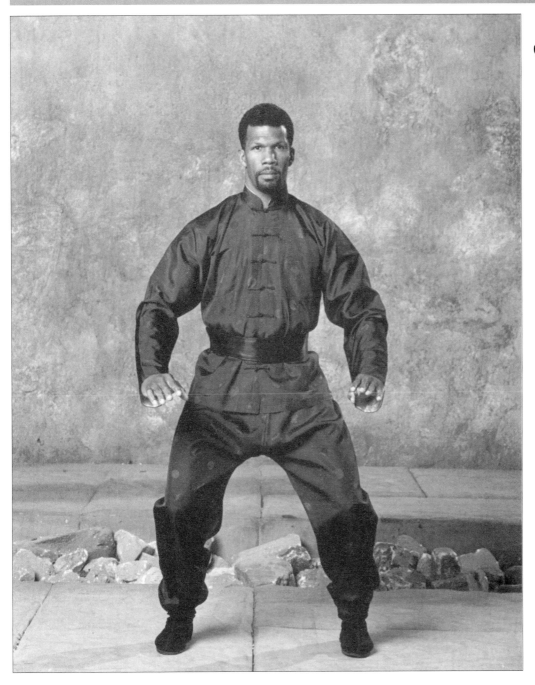

another. Slightly bend your knees as you raise your hands. Now lower your hands, turning the wrists so the palms are facing downwards. As you drop your hands bend your knees a little more. Raise your hands to shoulder level again, straightening your legs a little, and repeat.

Relax and move as if you are suspended in water.

太極計划

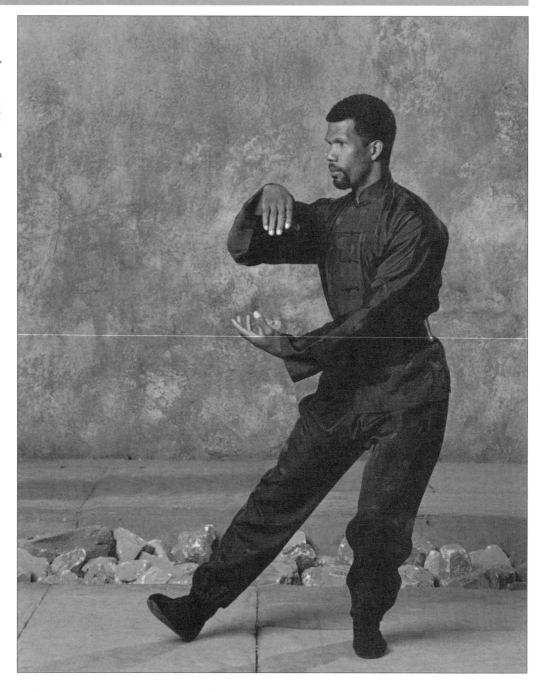

Hold the Ball

Start in a Right Heel Stance. Hold your left arm in an arc in front of your body, with the palm facing upwards, and your right arm forming an arc over the top, palm facing downwards. Imagine that you are massaging a beach ball, with both hands circulating, clockwise, keeping your palms facing one another. If you relax your right arm the elbow will bend as you bring your hand towards your body.

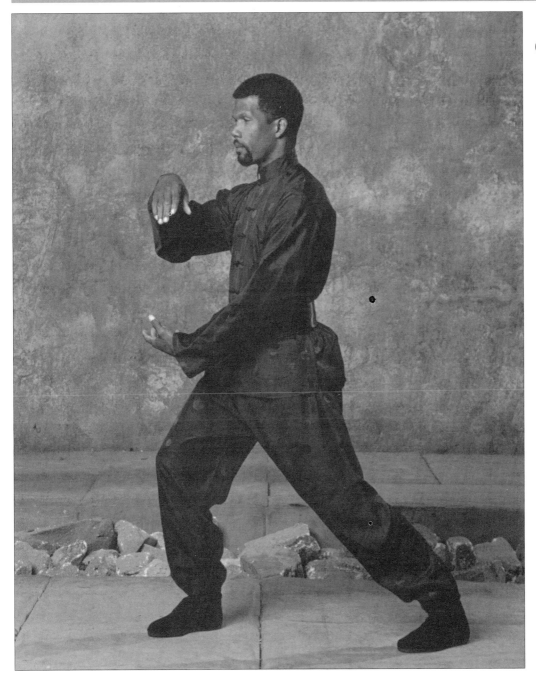

When your hands are away from your body, shift the weight forward onto your right foot and as your hands come in to your body, shift the weight back to your left foot. Allow your torso to rotate naturally as you move.

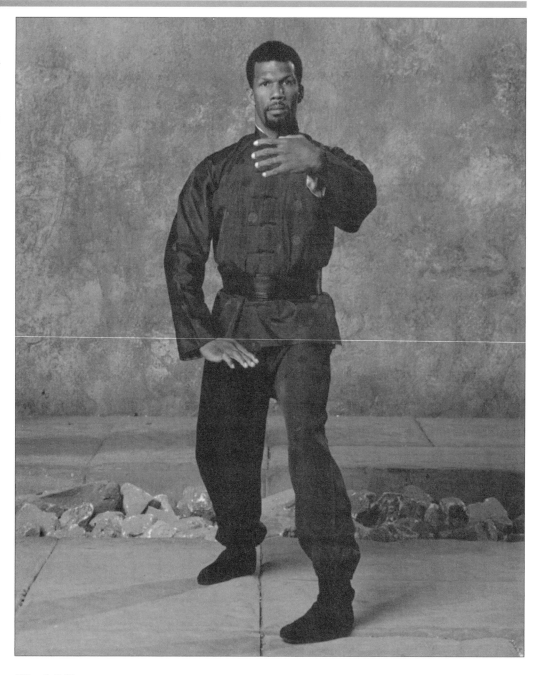

太極計划

Ward Off

Start in a Left Forward Stance with your hands crossed just in front of your chest, palms facing towards your chest. Push your left arm out in front of your body and raise it to shoulder level as though you are pushing someone with your forearm. At the same time, push your right arm downwards in an arc towards your right hip. Then bring your left arm in to your left shoulder and push it down in an arc towards your hip, and at the same time push your right arm out in front of your body in an arc, raising it to shoulder level. As you push your right palm down, it should face downwards, as the left palm ascends it should face your body, and vice versa. As your left hand reaches shoulder level, shift your weight backwards, and when your right hand reaches shoulder level, shift your weight forwards. Keep circling and allow your torso to rotate as you move. Relax.

That which shrinks
Must first expand.
That which fails
Must first be strong.
That which is cast down
Must first be raised.
Before receiving
There must be giving.

This is called perception of the nature of things.
Soft and weak overcome hard and strong.

Fish cannot leave deep waters,
And a country's weapons should not be displayed.

Lao Tsu

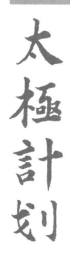

The ancient masters were subtle, mysterious, profound, responsive.

The depth of their knowledge is unfathomable.

Because it is unfathomable,

All we can do is describe their appearance.

Watchful, like men crossing a winter stream.

Alert, like men aware of danger.

Courteous, like visiting guests.

Yielding, like ice about to melt.

Simple, like uncarved blocks of wood.

Hollow, like caves.

Opaque, like muddy pools.

Who can wait quietly while the mud settles?

Who can remain still until the moment of action?

Observers of the Tao do not seek fulfilment.

Not seeking fulfilment, they are not swayed by desire for change.

Lao Tsu

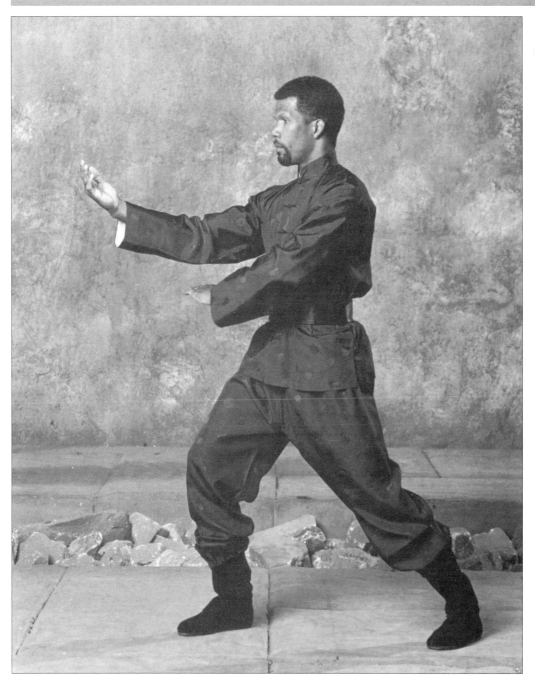

Back Palm

Start in a Right Forward Stance, with your hands crossed just in front of your body, palms facing inwards. Both hands circle away from your body. First, circle the right arm forward away from your body, keeping the palm facing you. At the same time, circle your left arm in a larger circle out to your left side, the palm always facing downwards. Both hands circle away from your body. You are pressing down with your left hand and back palming with your right.

73

太極計划

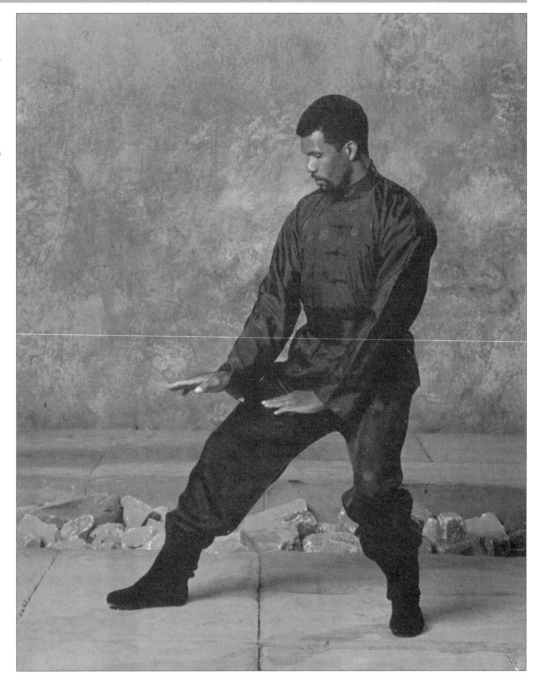

Rollback-Double Push

Start in a Right Forward Stance, with your hands held naturally by your sides. Pull your hands inwards, with the palms facing downwards, in an upwards arching motion. Shift your weight back to the left foot as your hands pull in as if you were pulling on a rope. Then, shift your

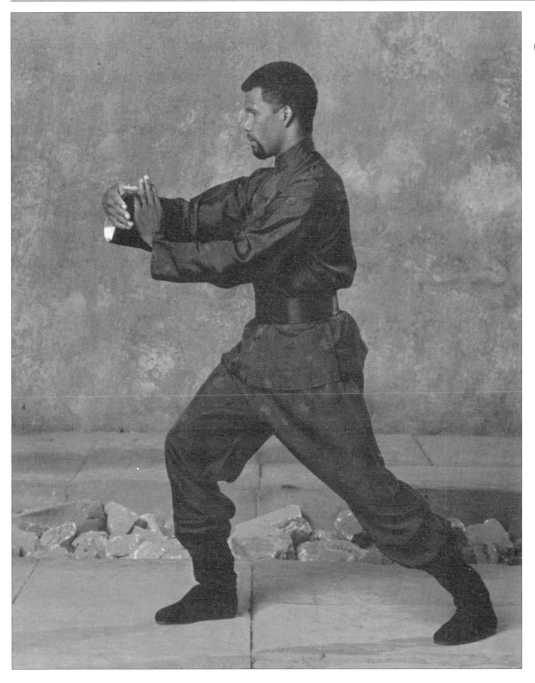

weight forward onto your right foot. As you do, push
your hands out in front with your right palm facing

inwards towards your body, and the side of your left hand
facing your palm. Your hands should travel in a full circle.

太極計划

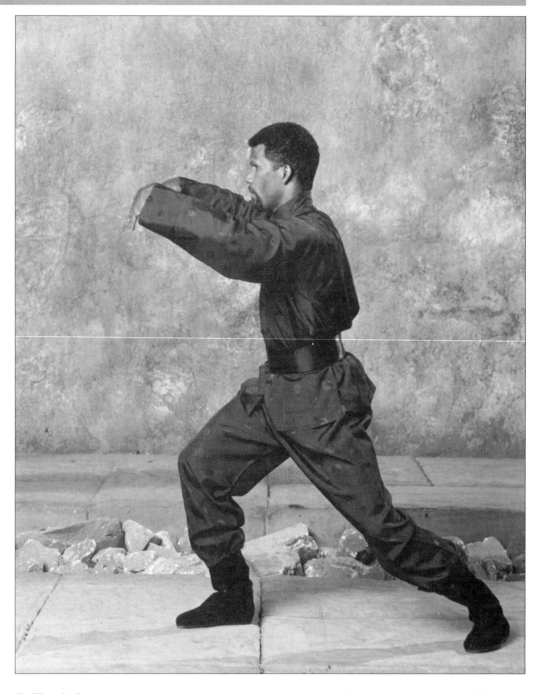

Rollback-Press

In a Right Forward Stance hold both hands in front of your body just below shoulder height, with the palms facing

down. Pull your hands back towards your head. They should pass either side of your head and brush by your ears as they go. Your hands then push away from your

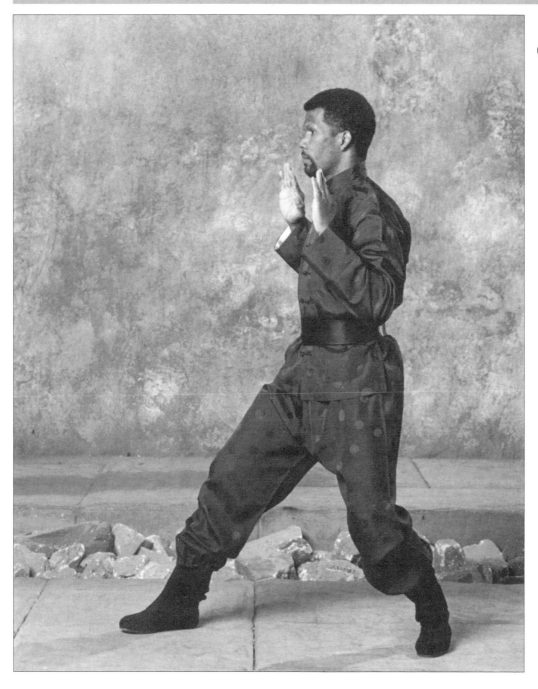

body with the palms facing forward. Your hands should travel in a continuous circle. As you pull backwards, shift back into a Right Heel Stance, and as you push forwards, shift into a Right Forward Stance.

Let the easy, slow movements release the tension from the moving body parts. Release any negative thoughts and anxiety.

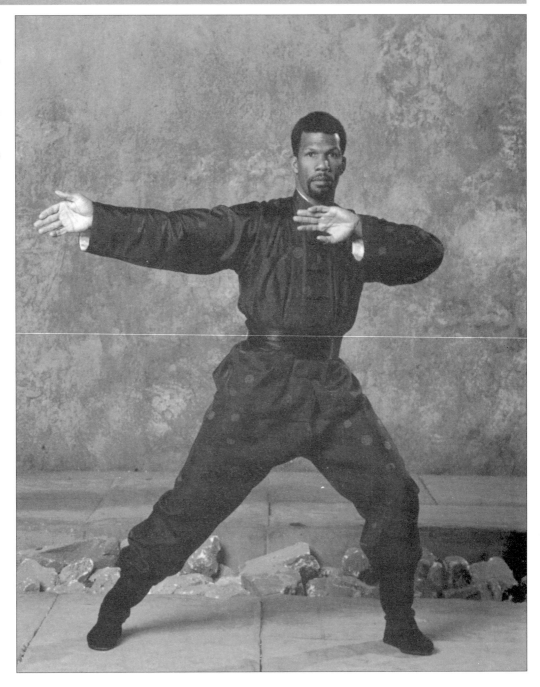

Sweeping Hands

Start in a Right Forward Stance with your right arm outstretched to the side at shoulder level and your left arm bent into your chest also at shoulder level. Your left hand should be twisted to face away from your body and the right palm should face the same direction. Sweep your arms across and outwards, bringing your right arm into your chest, and outstretching the left to the side.

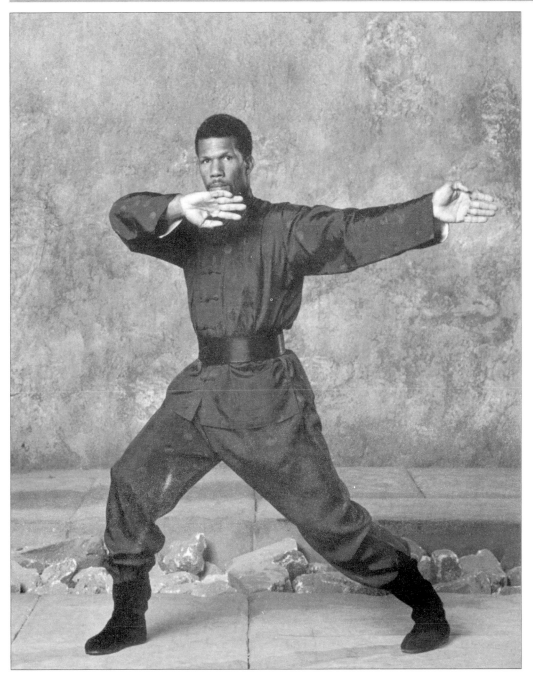

Twist your hands so that the palms still face outwards. As you sweep across you should transfer your weight to your left leg and twist your feet to the left, into a Left Forward Stance. Continue by shifting back and forth between Left and Right Forward Stance as you sweep your arms. Allow your torso to move from side to side naturally. Get the whole body into the move, relax and feel the air pushing the palms back as they sweep.

太極計划

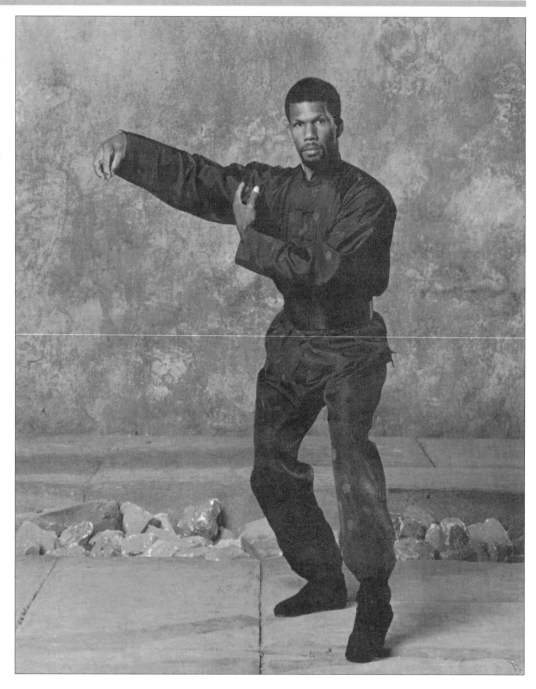

Outer Foot Block

Start in a Left Cat Stance with your left arm bent and held across your chest and the palm facing your right shoulder. Your right arm is held up at shoulder level and bent at the elbow. The wrist should be bent forward and the fingers and thumb bent together as if you were holding something in your finger tips, forming a 'Crane's Beak'. Lift your left leg bending your knee and kick your

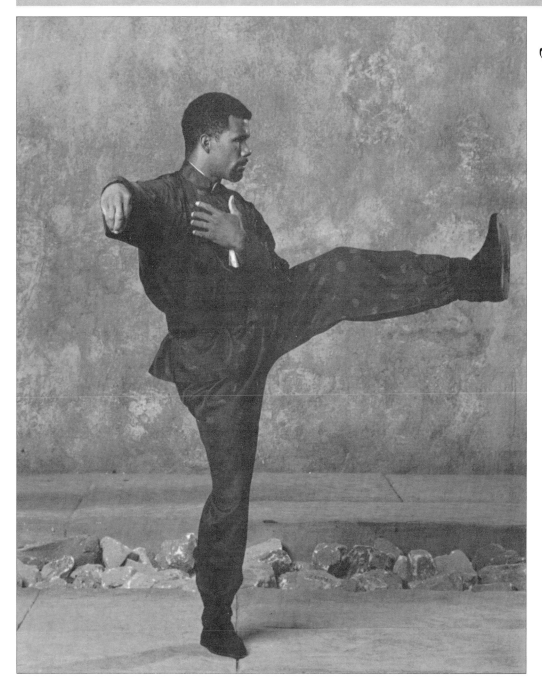

leg outwards, towards the left in a circling motion. Keep your weight on your right leg so that your left leg remains light and relax your right foot for greater balance. Relax as you throw the kick. Do not force out the power and speed, it has to come naturally, if you are tired and hurting then stop and continue later. Let endurance and strength develop naturally.

太極計划

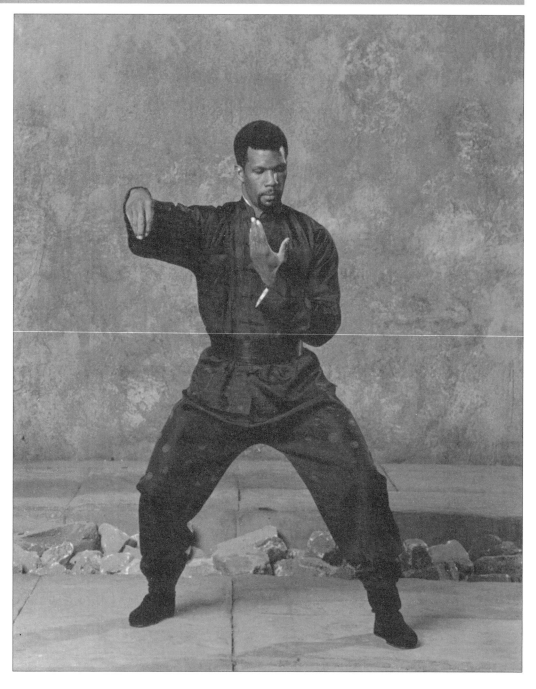

Guide In-Push Out

Start in a Left Heel Stance with your right arm held out at shoulder level, bent at the elbow, and the hand held in a Crane's Beak position. Fold your left arm into your chest, with the palm facing your body. Arc your left hand outwards from the centre of your body, in a circular direction, with the palm facing outwards. As your arm turns to travel towards you the palm should turn to face your body. Your left hand should now have travelled in a full circle. When it returns to your chest, push it forwards,

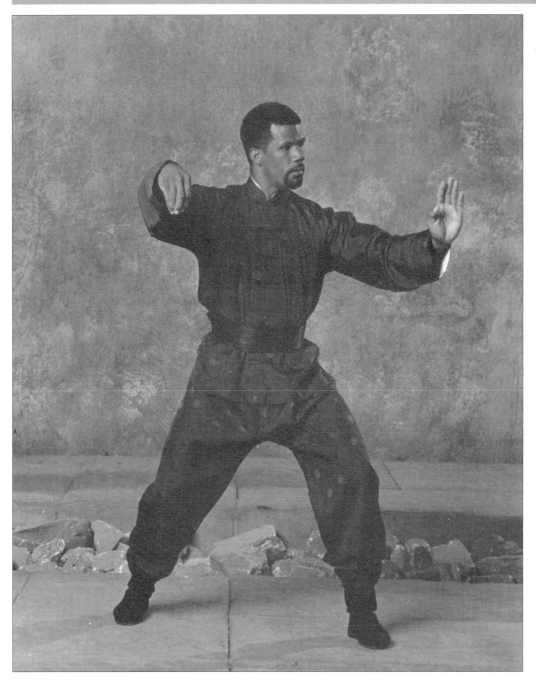

with the palm facing forwards, in an upwards arching motion. This hand should travel a full circle and a half. As you move your upper body, co-ordinate your stance positions. When the left hand is by your chest, lean back into Left Heel Stance. When your hand is outstretched move into Left Forward Stance.

All of the movements are connected. The moves of the arms, torso and hands are directly influenced by the leg and feet movements. Breathe deeply and evenly. Use your breathing to relax.

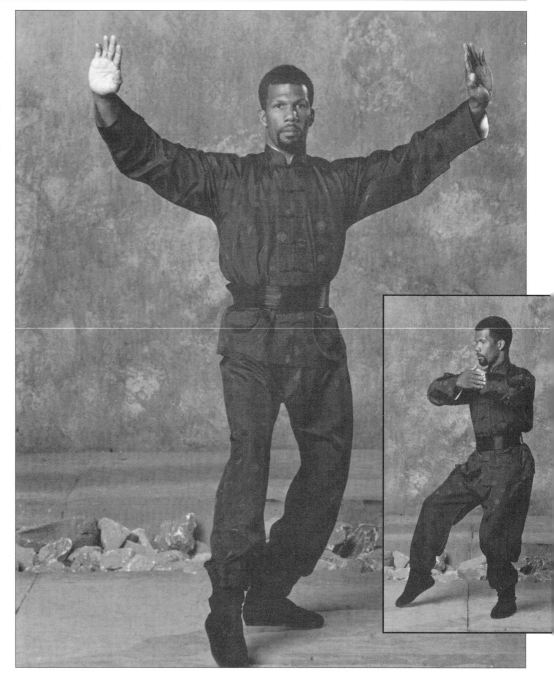

Spread the Wings

Start from a Right Cat Stance, with your arms crossed in front of your chest. Raise both hands upwards, to above the head and then lower your hands outwards down

either side of your body, forming a large circle. Bend at the waist, so that the circle reaches the knees. As you rise up from the bend, cross your arms in front of your body. Once you are standing straight again, and your arms are

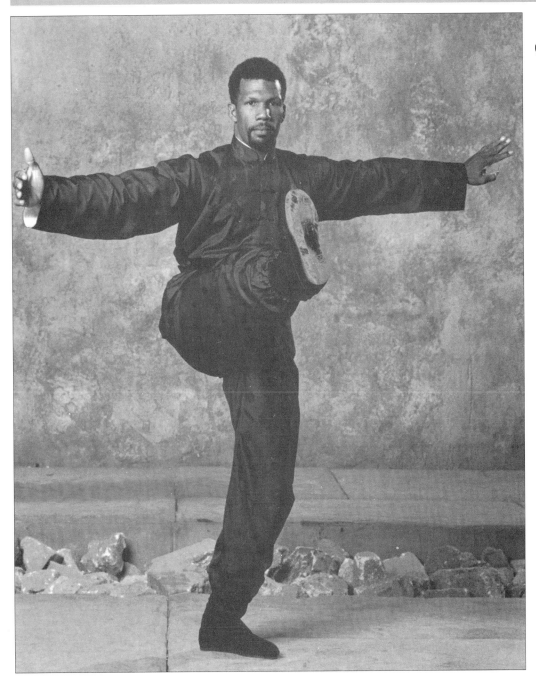

crossed, twist your torso to the left from the hips so that your right hand lies across your body. Lift your right leg, bending at the knee and kick your leg in an outwards arching motion towards your right. At the same time, fling your arms outwards, allowing the back of your right hand to slap the inside of your right foot as it kicks out. You should come back to a cat stance and bring your arms into the body to begin the move again.

太極計划

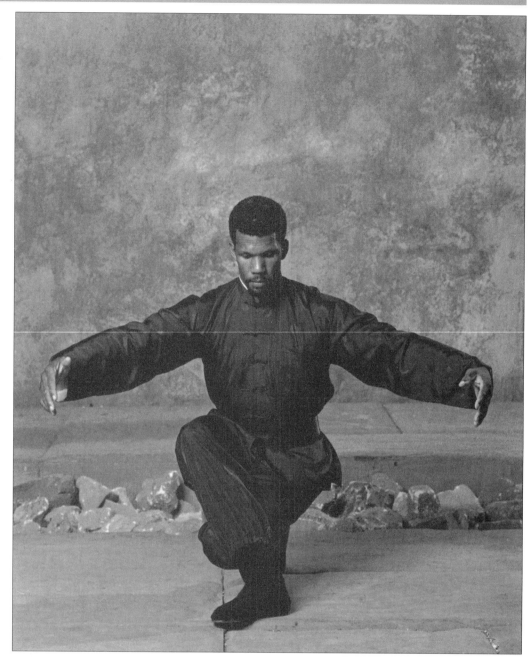

Gather the Leaves

Start in a Right Cross Stance, with your arms outstretched at shoulder level on either side of your body and with your fingers facing downwards. Lower your hands on either side of your body, bending at the knees and the waist to lower your stance. As you bend your knees, bring your hands round to cross just before your right leg in front, as if scooping up leaves. Imagine you are gathering energy. As you straighten your legs, bring your hands up, crossed, to your mid section. Then open up your hands, spreading your arms out to the side again and raise them to be level with your head. Now, repeat the move.

Do not let your weight fall forward, keep it centred at all times, and keep your back straight. This will strengthen the thighs, hips and buttocks.

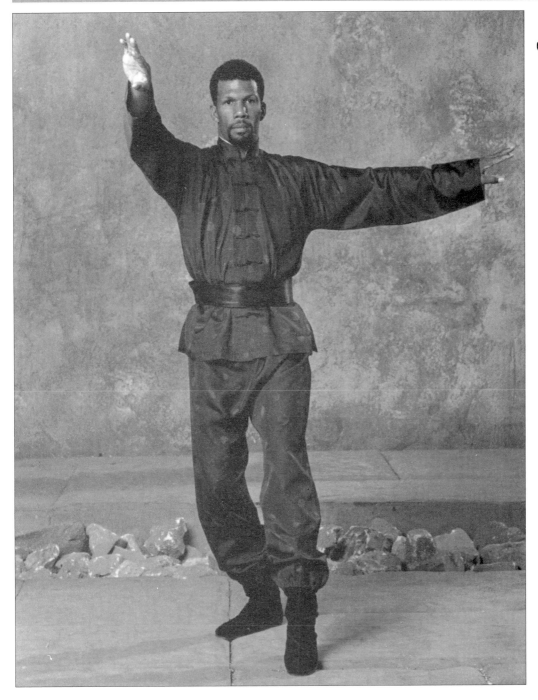

Wrist Rotations

Start in a Left Cat Stance with your left arm outstretched at shoulder level directly to the left side. The right arm should be outstretched slightly forwards, so that your hand is held above your head. Rotate your hands from the wrists towards your body three times. Then rotate the hands away from your body three times. As you rotate, relax your knees so that you bend slightly, in rhythm with the rotations. Relax the shoulders. Pull your energy up from your legs, through your hips, back, shoulders, arms, elbows and wrists to your fingertips. Feel the energy flowing through every part of your moving body.

87

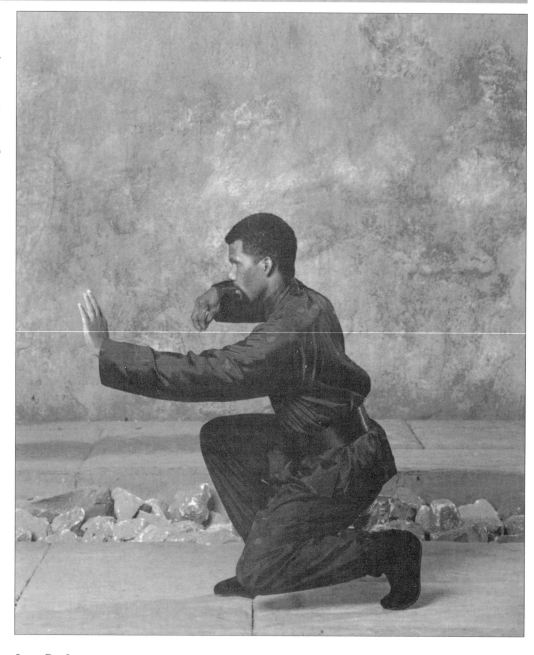

太極計划

Low Push

Start in the Left Cat Stance with your left arm outstretched at shoulder level to the side, and the right arm outstretched slightly in front, above head level. Form a Crane's Beak with your right hand, and hold this at shoulder level throughout the move. You will turn your whole body 180° to finish in a right kneeling stance. Turn to your right and lower your stance into the kneeling position. As you do, sweep your left hand past your left ear and push forward. The move should finish with your right foot in front of your left, with both knees bent and your left hand striking forward. Hold for a few seconds before beginning the move again. Keep your spine as straight as possible.

No matter how complicated the move seems at first, remember to concentrate on relaxing the body. If you are relaxed the body will naturally align itself.

In the pursuit of learning, every day something is acquired.

In the pursuit of Tao, every day something is dropped.

Less and less is done

Until non-action is achieved.

When nothing is done, nothing is left undone.

The world is ruled by letting things take their course.

It cannot be ruled by interfering.

Lao Tsu

太極計划

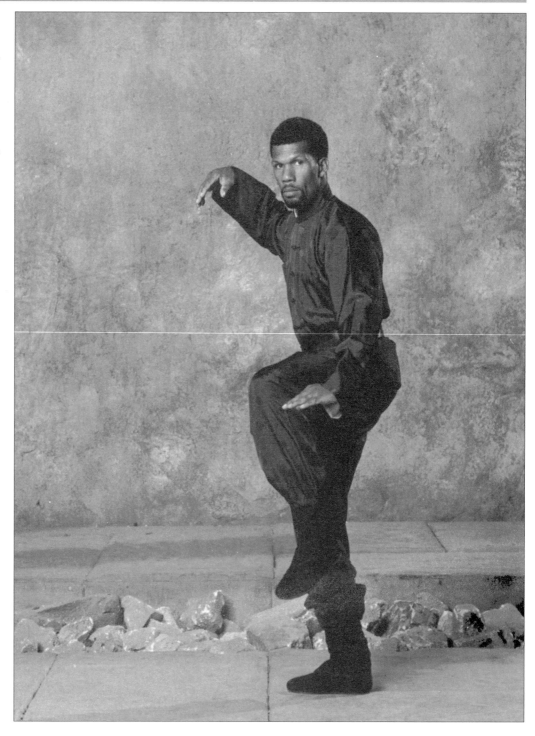

Brush Knee-Push

Start in a Left Cat Stance with your left hand held in front of your forehead, with your palm facing outwards, and your right hand in the Crane's Beak position held out at your side. Raise your left knee into a Left Crane Stance. As you raise your knee, lower your left hand, with the palm facing downwards, across your body and in front of your knee. This is a low block. Then step into a Left

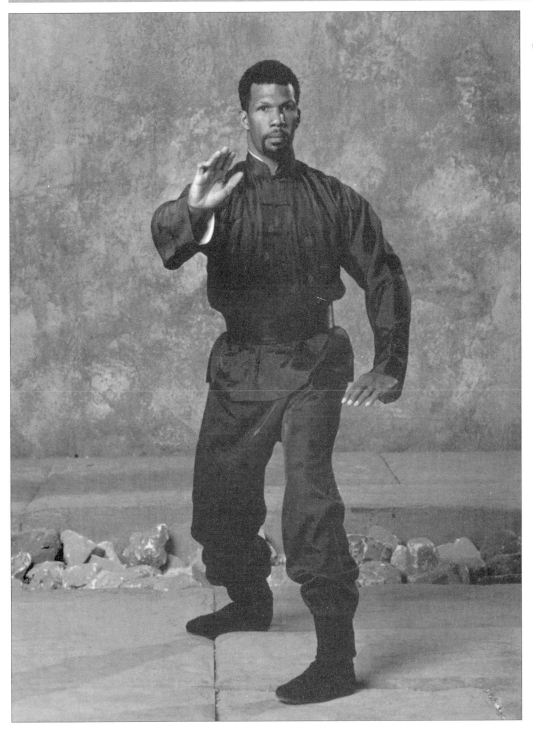

Forward Stance. As you shift your weight forwards, push your right hand to the front in an arching motion with your palm facing ahead. Rotate your hips so that you are facing forwards.

Remember, when you breathe keep the tip of your tongue on the roof of your mouth. This allows you to breathe deeper. The tongue serves as a connector for the chi flow within the body.

91

太極計劃

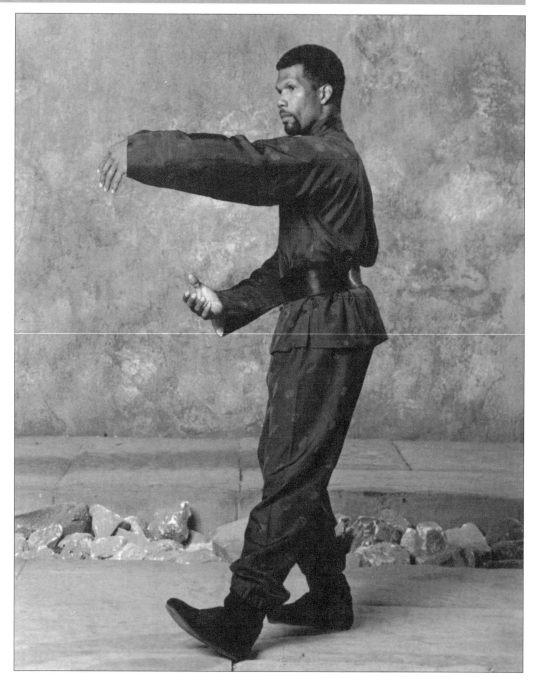

Play the Guitar

Start in a Horse Stance and turn 45° to your left, into a Left Heel Stance. As you turn, pull your left hand across the mid section of your body, in an arching motion, and allow your right hand to follow. The palms should be facing one another. Push both hands forwards, with the

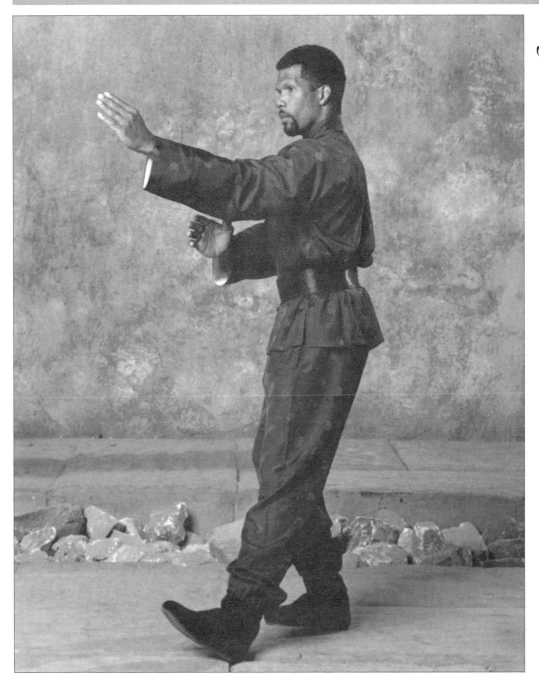

left palm facing your body with the side of your right hand facing the left palm, thus pushing your left hand slightly further. Relax into the stance and hold, before returning to horse stance to repeat.

Let go of any outside thoughts. The more the mind relaxes, the more efficiently it works. The muscles relax and the mind is calm.

太極計划

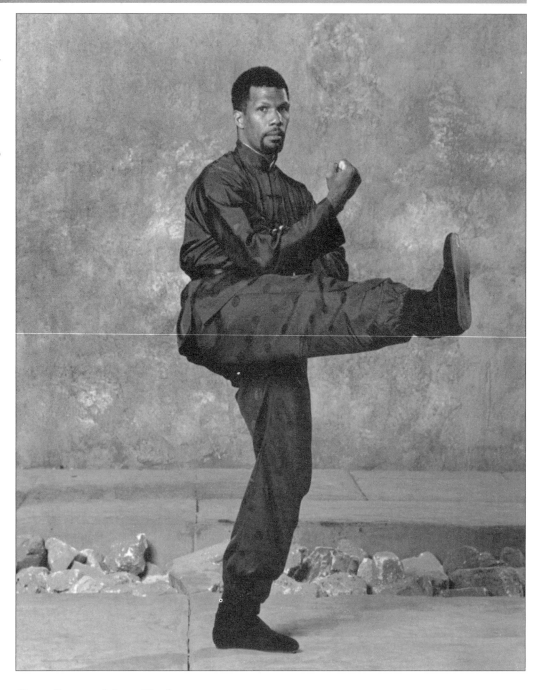

Outer Foot and Arm Block

Start in a right cat stance, with your left arm bent at the elbow and held naturally next to your body, and your right arm bent at the elbow, the forearm held in front of your chest. Clench your right hand into a fist. Raise your right leg bending at the knee and kick in an arching motion outwards towards the right. As you kick, arc the right arm outwards leading with the back of the fist. The arm and leg should make the same arc, at the same time. Keep the weight back on your left leg. Do not force the kick too high, too fast.

94

Returning is the motion of the Tao.

Yielding is the way of the Tao.

The ten thousand things are born of being.

Being is born of not being.

Lao Tsu

太極計划

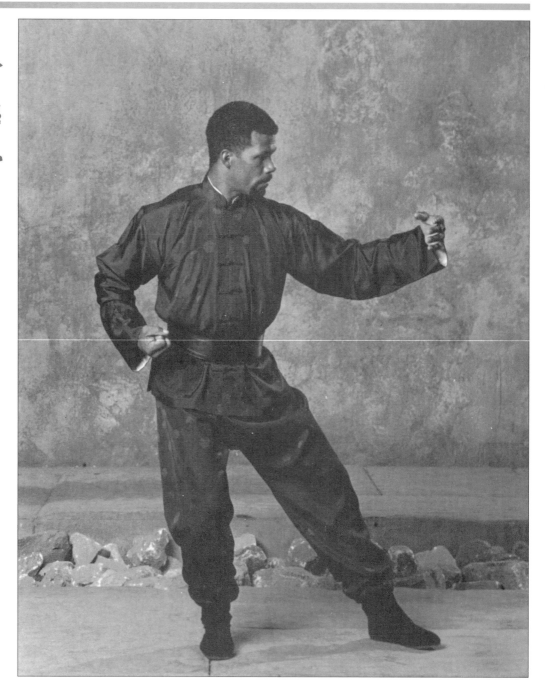

Punch

Start in a Left Forward Stance with your right hand held in a fist by your right hip and your left hand held in front with the palm facing your body. Punch with your right fist, in a circular motion, arching upwards from the hip to punch forward. Allow your left hand to cover your right as it arcs downwards in the opposite direction towards the body. Then, complete the circle by bringing your right fist in an arching downwards motion towards your body. Your left hand does the opposite and arcs upwards

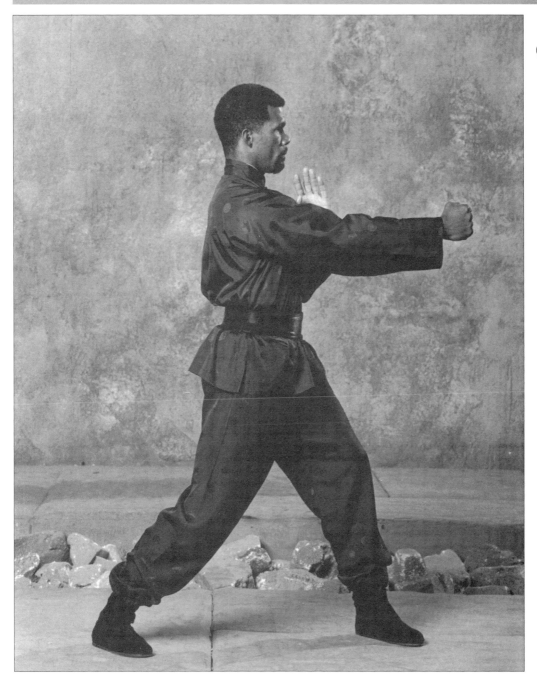

and away from your body. As you punch forwards, your weight should be forward on your left foot, with your hips rotating slightly. As you pull back, your weight should be centred.

The energy starts in the feet, transfers to the waist which rotates the torso, transferring to the shoulders, arms, and finally the fists. The power of the move involves the entire body.

太極計划

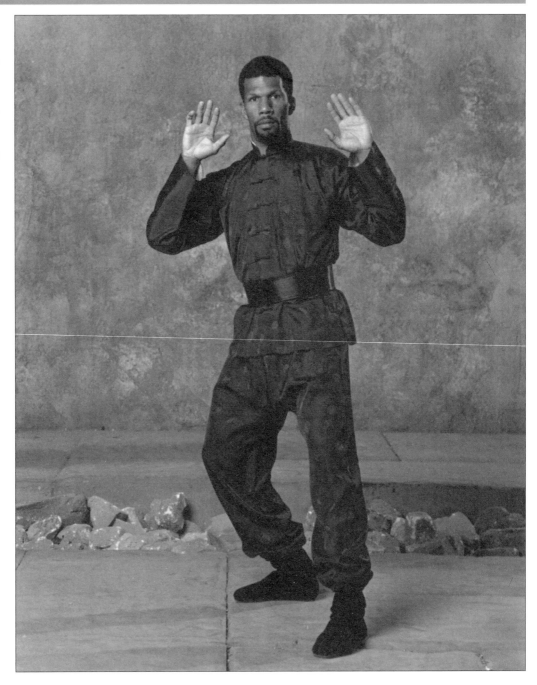

Rollback-Double Push

Start in a Left Forward Stance with your hands crossed in front of your chest and both palms facing your body. Pull both hands towards you, passing either side of your head at ear level. As they reach your ears, push your hands down and away from you keeping them at shoulder level. Keep your hands facing the same direction, so that the palms face forwards when you push out. As you pull back, drop back into a Left Heel Stance. As you push out, shift to a Left Forward Stance.

Stay in balance. Relax and feel the energy push out from your fingers.

Between birth and death,

Three in ten are followers of life,

Three in ten are followers of death,

And men just passing from birth to death also number three in ten.

Why is this so?

Because they live their lives on the gross level.

He who knows how to live can walk abroad

Without fear of rhinoceros or tiger.

He will not be wounded in battle.

For in him rhinoceroses can find no place to thrust their horn,

Tigers no place to use their claws,

And weapons no place to pierce.

Why is this so?

Because he has no place for death to enter.

Lao Tsu

太極計划

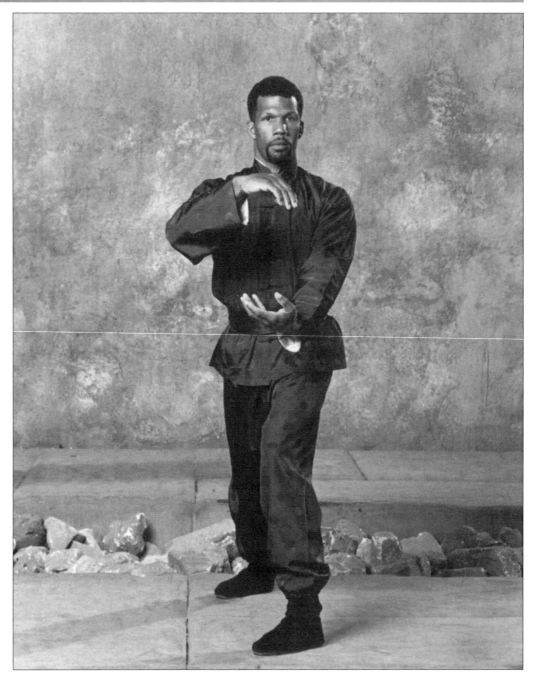

Spread the Arms

Start in Left Forward Stance with both hands outstretched in front with the palms facing one another, and your weight forwards. Turn to the right, and as you do, move your left arm above the right, into Holding the Ball. As you turn 45°, keep your hands turning so that they cross

100

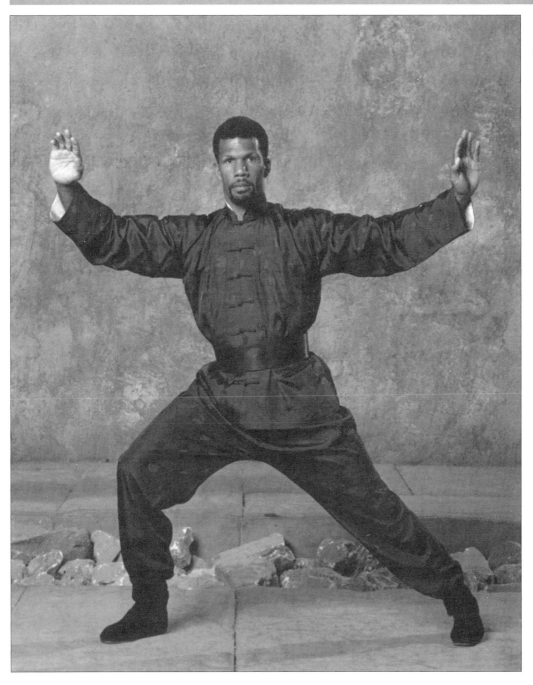

in front of your face, open your hands outwards to
extend either side of your body to shoulder level. You
should finish in a Right Forward Stance.

太極計划

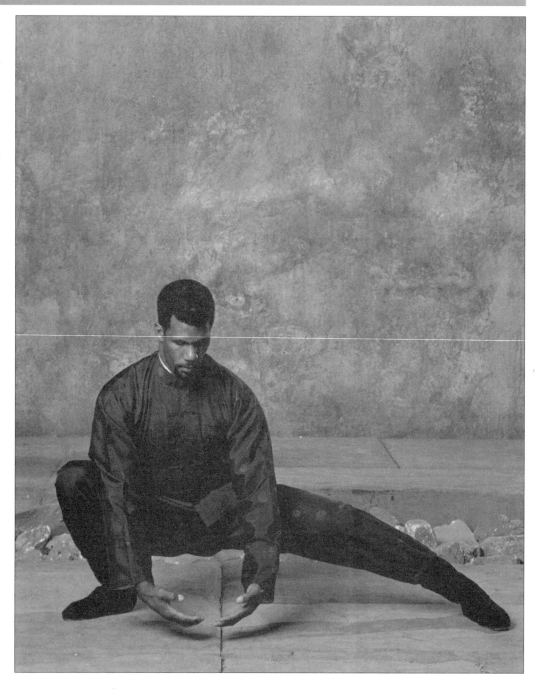

Polk Stance-Finish

From a Horse Stance, drop to a Right Polk Stance with your hands outstretched to the sides. Then bring your hands in towards your body so that your hands cross. Scoop up your hands and stand up raising them to your chest. Once standing gradually push your hands down

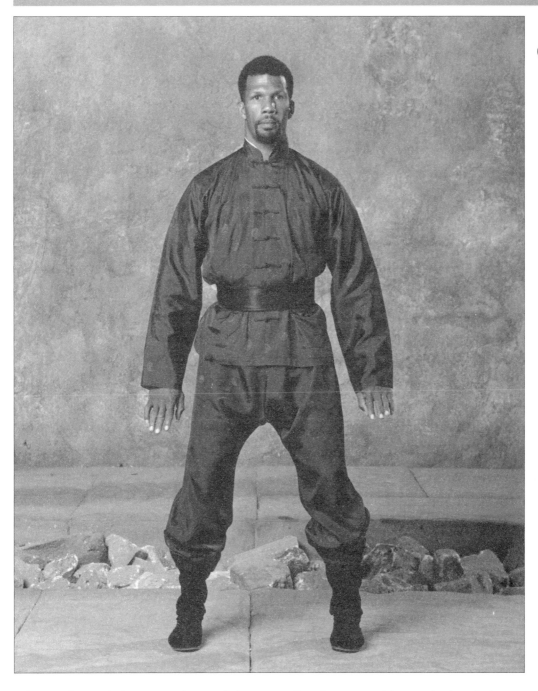

either side of your body, keeping your fingers pulled back.

Try to keep your weight centred and your back straight throughout, and relax.

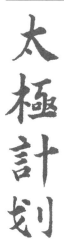

THE COMPLETE FORM

Before you attempt to do the entire form, make sure you are comfortable with the individual moves, so that you already know the moves, and you just need to learn The Transitions.

Try to combine one new move with the moves you have already learned every day. Build up the form like adding links to a chain.

Make sure you are in balance at all times when flowing from move to move. Once you know the entire form, try to do the form as slowly as possible. It should take about three to four minutes. Try to work on the form for thirty minutes but if you have little time then do it at least once.

The Chinese philosopher Lao Tsu once said, 'nothing is weaker than water, but when it attacks something hard or resistant then nothing withstands it and nothing will alter its way'. Tai Chi works the same way, the power of Tai Chi comes from a constant flow of motion, each successive move adds more power to the next move. The body parts travel in a spherical trajectory so that no energy is wasted. Let go and allow the naturalness of the moves to flow together. The complete form is performed without stops or breaks. The body never stops moving, the energy never stops flowing.

The Transitions

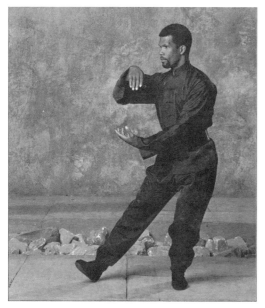

1 From the Opening Move rotate your body to your right. Shift 80% of your weight to your left leg and form a Right Heel Stance. Your arms should form the second posture, Do one rotation of Hold the Ball.

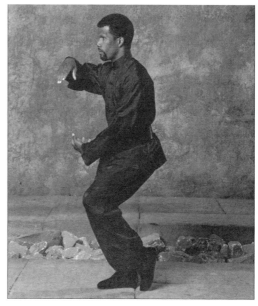

2 Shift all of your weight to your right foot. Push your left toe forward so that it is in front of your right foot. Then step forward into a Left Forward Stance.

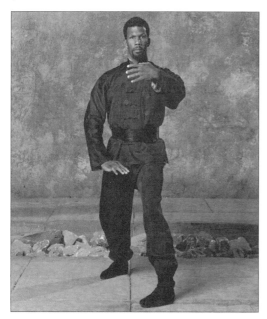

Push your right hand forwards in an arching motion and then allow it to glide down to your right hip. At the same time pull your left hand upwards into a Ward Off position.

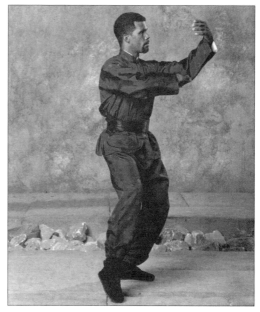

3 Hold your hands at face level with the palms facing one another, as if you are holding a ball. Turn your left foot 45° outward. Shift all of your weight onto your left foot. Bring your right foot in at a 45° angle to the right of your left foot. You should be in a Right Cat Stance.

太極計劃

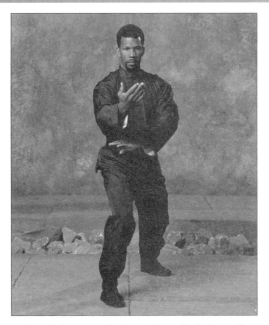

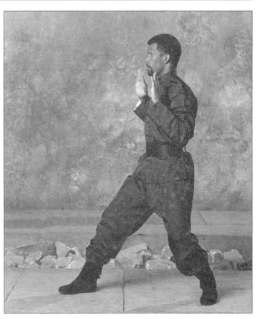

4 Now shift your weight forward into a Right Forward Stance. Execute the Back Palm. You should be at a 45° angle from your starting position to the right.

5 In the same stance execute a Rollback-Double Push.

6 Still in the Right Forward Stance, relax the arms so that they drop down to beside the waist. Then pull the hands up into Rollback-Press.

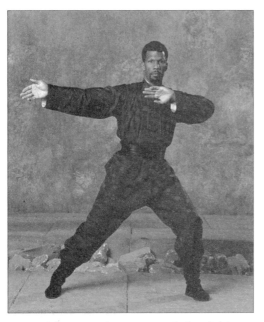

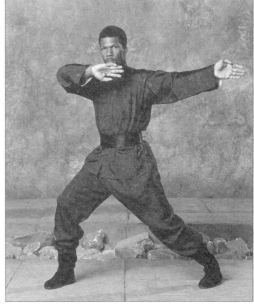

7 Now shift your weight up to your right foot, lightly move your left foot forward so that it is parallel to the right. Both feet should face forward. Now shift your weight to the left into a Left Forward Stance and execute Sweeping Hands.

Shift back to the right and sweep back, finishing in a Right Forward Stance.

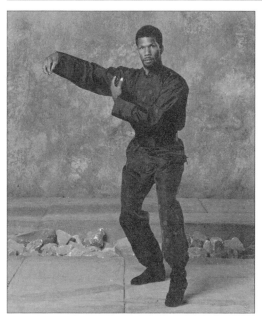

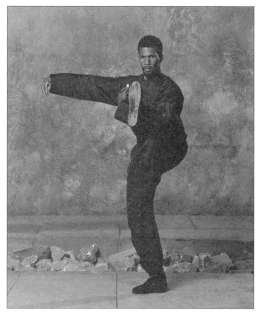

8 Slightly turn your right foot towards the left. Turn your torso to the left. Pull your left toe in to form a Left Cat Stance.

Execute the Outer Foot Block.

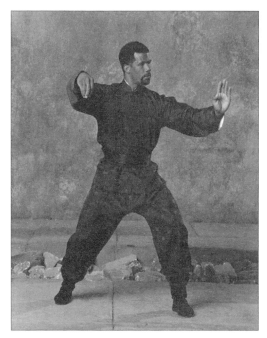

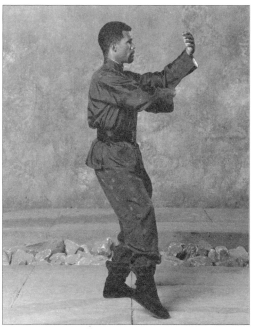

9 Shift your weight forward into a Left Forward Stance. Perform Guide In-Push Out finishing in a Left Forward Stance.

10 Rotate your left foot out to the left and shift all your weight on to it. Rotate your torso to the left and bring your right foot up, in front of the left into a Right Cat Stance. Execute Spread the Wings.

太極計划

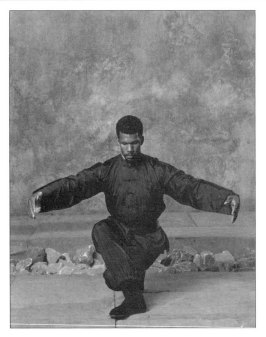

11 After you kick, let your right foot land directly in front of you. Turn your right foot 90° out to the right and slide your left knee up behind your right knee. Drop into a Cross Stance and then Gather the Leaves.

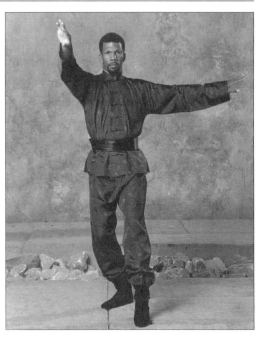

12 Bring your left foot forward into a Left Cat Stance. Do the Wrist Rotations.

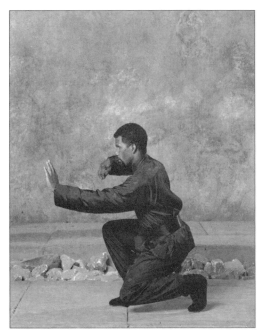

13 Turn 180° towards the right. Drop your weight equally between your legs and crouch into a Kneeling Stance. Execute the Low Push.

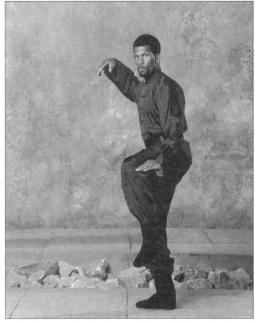

14 From the Kneeling Stance stand up and rotate your body 180° back to the left into a Left Cat Stance. You are facing the same direction as you were two moves ago. Lift your left knee and administer the Brush Knee-Push.

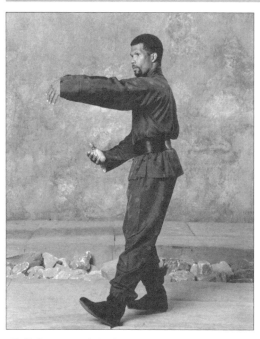

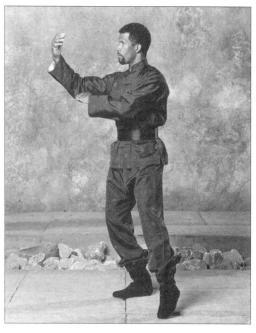

15 Shift your weight back to your right foot, move your left heel 45° to the right. Assume a Left Heel Stance and Play the Guitar.

16 Raise your hands in front of your face as if you were holding a ball. Turn to the right, lifting the left heel into a cat stance.

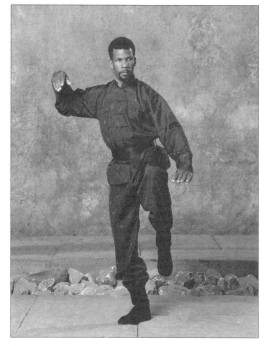

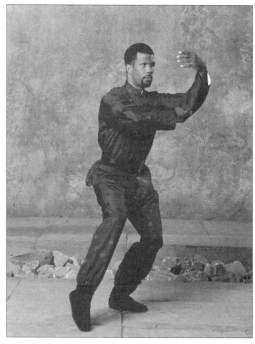

As you execute BrushKnee-Push, turn 45° to the left.

17 Execute another Brush Knee-Push 45° towards the right.

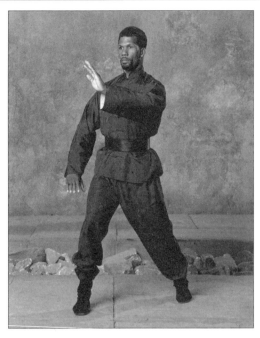

18 Again, do another Brush Knee-Push, 45° towards the left.

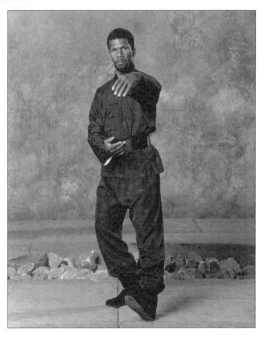

19 Shift your weight back to the right foot, move your left heel 45° to the right to 'square up' your Left Heel Stance. Perform Play the Guitar.

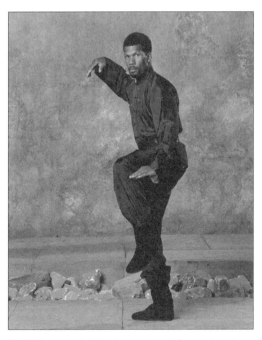

20 Shift your weight back to your right foot and again, perform Brush-Knee Push.

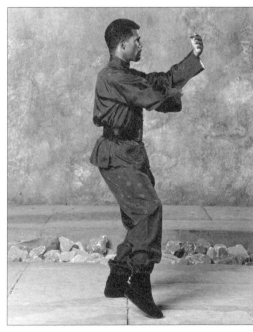

21 Shift your weight forward to your left foot. Bring your right foot forward, in front of your left foot and turn to the left, you should be in a right cat stance. Execute the Outer Foot and Arm Block.

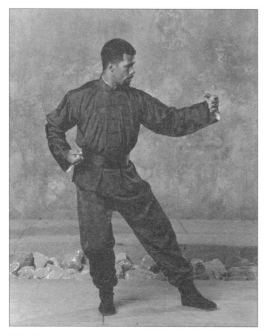

22 After you kick let the right foot land next to the left foot. Step forward with your left foot into a Left Forward Stance. Execute a Punch.

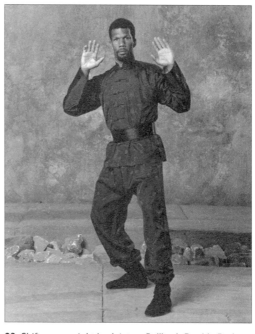

23 Shift your weight back into a Rollback-Double Push.

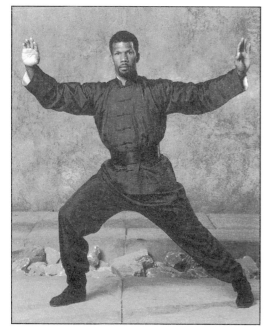

24 Turn to the right and shift your weight back to the right leg and Spread the Arms.

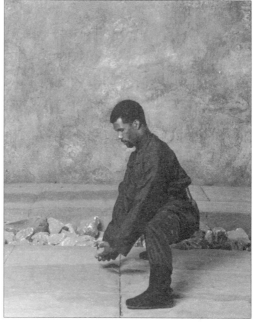

25 Let your torso drop down into the Polk Stance-Finish.

太極計划

Empty yourself of everything.
Let the mind become still.
The ten thousand things rise and fall while the Self watches their return.
They grow and flourish and then return to the source.
Returning to the source is stillness, which is the way of nature.

Lao Tsu

太極和你

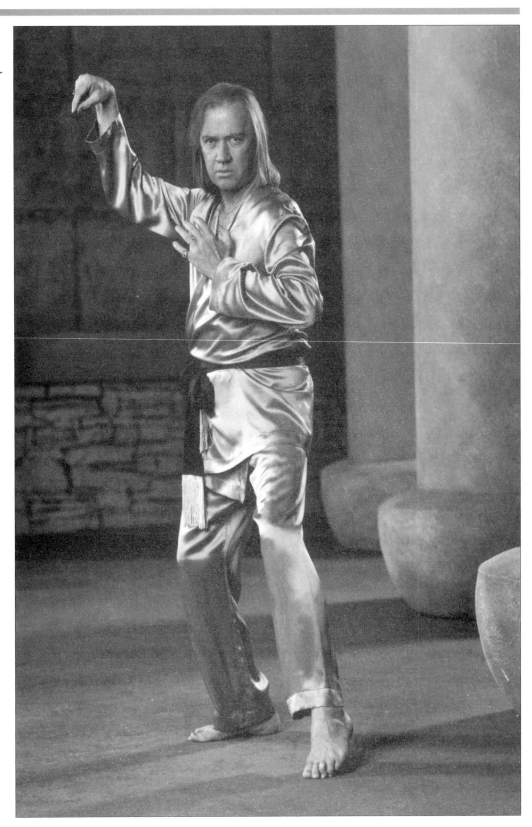

太極和你

Tai Chi and You

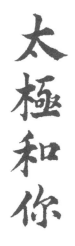

Practise non-action.
Work without doing.
Taste the tasteless.
Magnify the small, increase the few.
Reward bitterness with care.

See simplicity in the complicated.
Achieve greatness in little things.

In the universe the difficult things are done as if they are easy.
In the universe great acts are made up of small deeds.
The sage does not attempt anything very big
And thus achieves greatness.

Lao Tsu

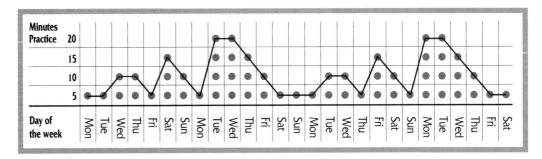

TAI CHI AND YOU

Chart Yourself

Often we stop doing beneficial things such as exercise, eating correctly and meditation, because we are not rewarded immediately. Conversely, if we feel better, we stop because we think we have solved the problem. It is recommended that you chart your progress on a calendar. Every day write down how many minutes you practise. Also write down anything else you did athletically or health-wise that is pertinent. Every time you enter a number you will feel good - it will reinforce your commitment, and give you a perception of your level of fitness. After 100 days or so, make a bar graph that corresponds to your minutes of practice.

Connect the points. Often you will see a wavy line, as opposed to a straight line of progression. This is completely natural. Since we are influenced by cosmic energies, biological energies, as well as busy schedules and personal demands, we cannot reasonably expect a straight line of progression. Fluctuation is completely natural.

Continue charting yourself see your progress over many months. You can also try comparing your chart to significant events in your life and see if there is a correlation.

116

Knowing harmony is constancy
Knowing constancy is enlightenment

Lao Tsu

Key to Success

The simple, most important factor in deriving any benefit from any self-development programme is 'consistency'. Total time, sweat, intensity, enthusiasm, intelligence, natural ability, pale in comparison to the importance of consistency. Let's compare the health of a person to a large wooden yoke resting on a pivot. The rotation of the yoke represents the natural flow of the health cycle. If we add energy to the system, the yoke turns. If we add energy everyday, we keep the yoke rotating. If we miss a day the yoke will stop. We then need a lot of energy to restart the rotation. If we spend most of our time stopping and restarting, we don't get very far.

Now imagine rain falling on the yoke. If the yoke is rotating the water will spin off and the wood stays healthy. If the yoke is still, the water seeps into the wood and dry rot occurs. Now a great amount of energy is needed to repair the wood instead of rotating the yoke.

You should do a basic five minutes every day, no matter what. Five minutes every day is much better than doing one hour three times a week. Try to do the five minutes in the morning because if you oversleep, then you have the chance to do the five minutes during your lunch break. If you cannot practise at lunch, then do five minutes after work; if this is not possible, then do five minutes after dinner. If not then, do five minutes before you sleep. The point being that it is best to do the minutes as early as possible so that you have plenty of opportunities to do them if you keep missing your set time. Once you get your basic five minutes out of the way, then pat yourself on the back. Try to do this for forty-five consecutive days. If you can do it for forty-five days in a row then you have created a habit for yourself. Soon you will 'want' to do it and no longer have to push yourself. Do not underestimate the accomplishment of doing five minutes every day for forty-five days. This could be the best thing you will ever do for yourself.

There are several exercises or sections in this book that can be recommended for the basic five minutes.

Any of the options can be done or interchanged daily, apart from meditation. However, five minutes is only a minimum, to avoid losing ground. Consult the Thirteen Week Programme, to find out how much time you should spend at each stage.

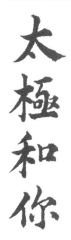

Option 1

Do the first five exercises of the Chi Kung section. This will stimulate your internal energy and lubricate the major joints of the body.

Option 2

Practise the Holding the Ball standing meditation exercise for five minutes. This will clear your mind, stimulate chi flow and develop strength in your back, legs, buttocks and arms. If you choose to do this then stick with it, as meditation is only effective if done consistently.

Option 3

As you are learning the individual Tai Chi moves, practise the move you are presently working on for five minutes.

Option 4

If you know all the moves, then do five moves for a minute each.

Option 5

If you know the entire continuous form then do it once, slowly.

Option 6

If you feel your legs are weak then do the Horse Stance, and the Left and Right Cat and Forward stances. Practise each posture for a minute.

Option 7

If you want an invigorating and intense five minutes of sweat and pain but great conditioning and an energy boost, then do a Low Horse Stance for five minutes. Try to get the thighs parallel to the floor and keep the back straight. Good luck. This is one of the most effective and efficient training methods in all of the Chinese martial arts.

The wise student hears of the Tao and practises it diligently.

The average student hears of the Tao and gives it thought now and again.

The foolish student hears of the Tao and laughs aloud.

If there were no laughter, the Tao would not be what it is.

Lao Tsu

INTEGRATE TRAINING INTO YOUR LIFE

There is nothing that can replace a good concentrated workout of meditation or Tai Chi. However, integrating Tai Chi exercises, the practice of meditation and Taoist philosophy into your whole life is just as beneficial and natural. You will find that there are precious hours even minutes in the day when you can meditate, exercise and release tension for even the basic five minutes. The idea is to steal a minute here and a minute there, as well as trying to practise your programme. It's like saving pennies, where every minute is a penny deposited, and another drop of chi added to your reservoir of vitality. After years of doing this, you will feel as if you have made the best investment of your life.

When sitting in a chair, at work or in the home, occasionally twist your torso and look behind you. This will keep the spine supple and release tension in the neck.

Whenever necessary, stretch your arms straight up in the air. Stretch with the same feeling as if you are waking up from a nap.

When you pick something up off the ground, bend at the waist, keep your back straight and knees locked.

When you brush your teeth, put your leg up on the counter, knee locked and bend at the waist towards your knee.

When you are really tired, lie down on your back, with your legs shoulder-width apart and arms down by your side. Make sure your body is in a straight line and symmetrical. Meditate. Lower your breathing, putting your tongue on the roof of your mouth and relax. You will either fall asleep or you will circulate the chi. Either is good.

In the same lying position, tense the buttocks and tighten the arms and then relax and repeat this several times. This is good stimulating chi flow, as it serves as a pump for the main chi cycle.

太極和你

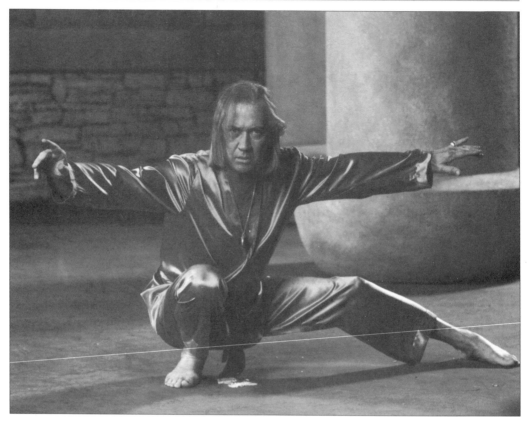

When you are sitting in a parked car, or as a passenger, in an office, or waiting for an aeroplane or bus, do a sitting meditation. Keep your back straight, feet flat on the floor, arms to your sides. Do not cross your arms or legs as this will inhibit chi flow. Breathe deeply and focus the awareness to the tan tien.

When you are walking, walk as if you have a plate on top of your head. This will align the body. Allow your arms swing freely and let the fingers naturally straighten. Put your tongue on the roof of your mouth and concentrate on the tan tien.

In sport, martial arts, and some performing arts, the initial method of learning is to mimic as exactly as possible the mechanics of the given art. The novice seeks to perform the steps correctly, to gain control over the body and to learn the rules. Once these mechanics are mastered, one is a novice no longer, and can now begin to develop an individual style. You can now begin to apply the underlying philosophy of Taoism, Tai Chi and Meditation to your own needs and creativity and devise a programme to suit your own lifestyle.

Your Tai Chi skill level will now not regress as long as you practise regularly. Unlike purely physical forms of exercise, Tai Chi can be enjoyed for the rest of your life.